KRAV MAGA

How to Defend Yourself against Armed Assault

KRAV MAGA

How to Defend Yourself against Armed Assault

Imi Sde-Or (Lichtenfeld), Founder of Krav Maga
Eyal Yanilov, Chief Instructor

Frog, Ltd.
Berkeley, California

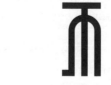

Dekel Publishing House
Tel Aviv, Israel

Krav Maga: How to Defend Yourself against Armed Assault

For information contact

Dekel Publishing House
P.O. Box 45094
Tel Aviv 61450, Israel.
www.dekelpublishing.com
ISBN 965-7178-00-2

Printed in Israel

Published in North America

by Frog, Ltd.
Frog, Ltd. books are distributed by
North Atlantic Books
P.O. Box 12327
Berkeley, California 94712
www.northatlanticbooks.com

Library of Congress Cataloging-in-Publication Data
Sde-Or (Lichtenfeld), Imi, 1910-1998
Krav Maga: How to Defend Yourself against Armed Assault / Imi Sde-Or (Lichtenfeld) and Eyal Yanilov
        p.   cm.
    ISBN 1-58394-008-1 (alk. paper)
    1. Self-defense--Israel.   I. Yanilov, Eyal, 1959-   .   II. Title.
GV1111.S38   2001
613.6'6'095694–dc21   9932767
                                                CIP

Dedicated to the blessed memory of my father and teacher, Samuel Lichtenfeld.

Imi Sde-Or (Lichtenfeld)

Si vis pacem para bellum.

If you want peace, prepare for war.

Krav Maga: *How to Defend Yourself against Armed Assault*

Technical Advisor & Professional Editor: Darren R. Levine

English Translation: Efrat Ashkenazi

Language Editor: Michelle Sachnin

Photography: Liat Paz

Photographs and drawings from Hebrew edition: Eldad Zakovitz

Further Photographs from Hebrew edition: Achihu Larom

Book Design: Rotem Namir-Pardess

Cover Design: Ayelet Yehuda, Nina Jawitz

Photo Prints: Studio Prior

Photo Scanning: Arad

Table of Contents

The significant contribution of the following Krav Maga organizations to the successful realization of this publishing project is greatly valued:

International Krav Maga Federation
Krav Maga Association of America
Israeli Krav Maga Association

The following instructors from the International Krav Maga Federation invested many hours, applying their expertise in demonstrating the various techniques in the 500-odd photographs contained in this volume. Their significant contribution to the coherence of this publication is greatly appreciated: **Gabi Noah**; **Eli Ben-Ami**; **Avi Moyal**; **Amnon Darsa**; **Dori Nemetsky**; **Yoav Gaon**. Thanks to the following Krav Maga instructors who feature in one or more of the historical photos contained in this book: **Shaike Barak**; **Hayim Zut**; **Guy Cohen**.

FOREWORD by the late Mr. **Yitzhak Rabin**

Dear Imi,

The imparting of physical fitness and Krav Maga to IDF soldiers and officers and Imi Lichtenfeld are one and the same, an integral part of IDF activity. My gratitude to you for your contribution to the Israel Defense Forces in cultivating "muscle-bound Judaism," and my congratulations on the publication of your book: a manual for moments of distress, in the hope that the readers will never have need for your advice and experience.

Sincerely,

Yitzhak Rabin

Prime Minister and Minister of Defense of Israel (written in 1992 for the original Hebrew-language edition)

FOREWORD by Mr. **Shimon Peres**

The two greatest dangers in the world today are war waged by missiles (and missiles do not respect borders), and knife fights (since terrorism does not respect borders either).

In war waged by missiles, technology is the decisive factor, and in terrorism, the individual. Imi Sde-Or, of blessed memory, developed a strategy for Krav Maga. A strategy that makes self-defense possible for the individual too, whether or not in uniform, such that even when alone on the battlefield, the battle will not necessarily be lost.

These days, with violence on the rise, this strategy is unparalleled.

Shimon Peres

Minister of Regional Cooperation,
and formerly Israel's Prime Minister

Acknowledgment

I wish to seize this opportunity to convey my gratitude to all those who were involved in the preparation of this book during the last few years, and especially to the following persons who played a crucial role in its realization:

Efrat Ashkenazi spared no effort in translating the Hebrew texts into fluent, everyday English (fortunately, her native language) and refining them over and over. **Liat Paz**, our photographer, was as patient as proficient with her camera, whether in her studio or outdoors and even posed for some of the hostage photographs. **Michelle Sachnin** worked indefatigably as language editor, doing her best to rescue the English text from our incessant "corrections." **Rotem Namir-Pardess**, who was responsible for the final form of the graphic design, did her job with impressive skill. **Uri Novojenov** took good care of the lab-work, providing us with the necessary printed photos that Liat has shot. **Chezi Mizrahi** exercised his professional talents to furnish us with quality scanning of the above photographs. **Dan Barkai**, pistol shooter and instructor, applied his expertise to ensure the accuracy of the information on firearms included in the book. **Abraham Lapidot** kindly furnished us with photographs of the various firearms needed for demonstration, by courtesy of Israel Military Industries (I.M.I.). And last but not least, **Judith Taffet**, secretary of Dekel, served as the coordinator responsible for this publishing project in Israel, and faithfully labored to ensure its successful culmination despite all difficulties and her many other duties.

And on the other side of the Atlantic Ocean:

Richard Grossinger, Publisher and President of Frog Ltd. and North Atlantic Books, who was the first American publisher to realize the ever-growing need for a comprehensive Krav Maga book on the US market, and boldly embarked on this Israeli-American publishing venture despite all difficulties. **Jess O'Brien**, Frog Ltd.'s Martial Arts Editor, made sure in his quiet and efficient way that everything was well integrated on the American end of the project, as well as providing us with his most helpful proofreading. **Nicole George** was most helpful in advising us on the correct rules of English punctuation. My personal friend and legal advocate, **Hugo Gerstl**, President and CEO of Four Paws Publishing, played a central role in realizing this publishing project while operating under both his professional hats, to find ingenious solutions for delicate legal subtleties. My colleague, **Iven Lourie**, President of Gateways Books & Tapes, had a central role in initiating this US-Israeli connection.

Special acknowledgment is made to the contribution of Mr. **Daniel Abraham**, a publicly spirited businessman, for his invaluable support in the early stages of introducing Krav Maga teaching into the United States.

Z. M.

Publisher's Preface

I do not usually write a foreword to the books I publish. This, however, is an unusual book by an unusual person.

Mr. Imi (Imrich) Sde-Or (Lichtenfeld), the renowned Israeli Grandmaster (1910-1998), was the creator of the acclaimed school of Krav Maga. Imi and his senior disciple and follower, Eyal Yanilov, spent more than a decade writing this series of books for the benefit of people the world over who may, in times of emergency, need this special knowledge.

Due to his vast knowledge and outstanding personality, Grandmaster Imi was regarded as a living legend by his numerous students and associates who respected him almost as a Guru. He created a modern self-defense discipline which embodies the central characteristics of his personality and reflects the events that shaped his fascinating life. Just like Imi himself, the Krav Maga method is logical, intuitive, direct, and practical, but most of all, sensitive and humanistic.

Imi Sde-Or drew on his exceptional understanding of the human body and human dynamics to establish a different system of self-defense and hand-to-hand combat. His extensive personal experience in real-life violent situations, as well as his knowledge of various fighting systems (including wrestling and boxing, in which he excelled in his youth), were ingeniously infused into Krav Maga. This fighting system was developed, tested, and improved during Imi's long career in the Israel Defense Forces, and later adapted to civilian life.

Despite his fierce appearance, Grandmaster Imi was never a warlike person, and he earnestly sought peace, which he considered to be the highest of all attainments. He always told his students that it is essential to excel in their Krav Maga training precisely so that they would not have to use excessive or unnecessary force, even in life-threatening situations. His greatest wish was that the teaching of Krav Maga would eventually evolve into an international brotherhood among its practitioners, bridging hatred, hostility and national boundaries.

Imi's Central European background also left its mark on the development of Krav Maga. Considering himself always a citizen of the world, and acting accordingly, Imi Sde-Or wished to transcend the narrow confines that characterized Krav Maga at its initial stage. Therefore, the new discipline reached beyond the Israel Defense Forces and was offered to civilian frameworks after it was tailored to meet their needs. As a result, Krav Maga is now regularly taught in Israel to classes of children, young people, men, and women, in private institutions as well as under the auspices of the Israeli Ministry of Education.

In recent years, the new discipline has extended far beyond the borders of Israel. There are now active Krav Maga clubs in the United States, in most European countries, in Brazil, Australia & New Zealand, and in other parts of the world. In some of these countries, Krav Maga was also formally adopted by government organizations and law-enforcement agencies and incorporated into their training curricula.

The Krav Maga series, whose publication commences with this book, aims to further broaden the audience of Krav Maga by making it accessible to professionals and to the general public outside Israel. It provides the reader with the essential tools for practicing Krav Maga, by teaching general principles and specific techniques which are explained in detail with the aid of over one thousand photographs and diagrams. The theoretical part presents relevant issues such as: principles behind the defense techniques, dealing with a violent incident, fighting tactics, training methods including mental training, safety in training, etc., plus useful appendices.

In short, this series constitutes the only authorized, comprehensive manual on Krav Maga ever written by its founder, Grandmaster Imi Sde-Or himself and his senior disciple and follower, Eyal Yanilov. It is recommended for the beginner, as well as the more advanced practitioner or instructor of Krav Maga who is already initiated into this discipline or into some other school of Martial Arts.

The present publication is the result of diligent teamwork by several dedicated individuals (see Acknowledgment). I would especially like to thank Darren Levine, Chairman of the Krav Maga Center in Los Angeles, for his prolonged, thorough, and careful work as technical adviser and professional editor of the English-language edition, without which this book would certainly have lacked its present clarity and style. I feel personally indebted to Eyal Yanilov, co-author of this book and Head Instructor of the International Krav Maga Federation, whose persistent efforts and determination over the past ten years, combined with his universally unmatched knowledge of this art, turned what seemed first but a vision into a reality.

On a personal note, I owe a lot to my family, and especially to my wife, Pnina, without whose encouragement and support I doubt if I could have ever coped with this demanding publishing project. Ilana Sde-Or, Imi's wife and companion for many years, was of great help in producing long-forgotten photos from Imi's past and some of his well-known sayings. Merav Yanilov-Hazan, Eyal's wife, immensely helped us with her juridical proficiency in various legal aspects of this publication.

Last but not least, my utmost reverence is to Imi, the creator of Krav Maga, an outstanding teacher, a true friend, and a great human being. We all miss him.

Zvi D. Morik, Publisher
Tel Aviv, January 2001

Introduction

The information provided in this book is comprised of original material from the comprehensive self-defense and hand-to-hand fighting system, known in Israel and worldwide by its Hebrew name: "Krav Maga" (contact fight). This unique method was originally developed in the Israel Defense Forces and various branches of the security services by its creator, Grandmaster Imi Sde-Or, and was later adapted to civilian needs as well. It is important to note that all the Krav Maga techniques have been thoroughly tested in real-life situations, improved upon and refined accordingly.

This is the first and only authorized manual of the Krav Maga discipline, written by its founder and his senior disciple. It comprehensively addresses defense techniques dealing specifically with an armed assailant who poses an imminent threat to the life of the defender or to the life of a third party. These state-of-the-art defensive tactics and techniques focus on an assailant armed with a sharp-edged weapon (such as a knife or a broken bottle), a blunt object (such as a stick or an iron bar), or a firearm (such as a handgun or a rifle). Other related subjects are also covered: using everyday objects as defensive weapons, neutralizing a handgun or a hand grenade threat directed at a third party in a hostage situation, special training methods used in Krav Maga (including mental training), and more.

As the scenarios addressed in this book deal primarily with an armed assailant, they are all potentially life-threatening situations. Whether one is faced with an aggressor wielding a large kitchen knife, a crowbar, or even a handgun, the lethal nature of the encounter requires an effective response. This response must be sound both physically and tactically in order to prevent serious bodily injury or, at worst, possible death. Therefore, the Krav Maga discipline combines mental, technical, tactical, and physical training in order to significantly increase one's chance to prevail even in the most dangerous of predicaments.

Krav Maga is a unique system that has received international recognition as an innovative, effective and highly practical self-defense and fighting method. This recognition has come largely from experts in Martial Arts and hand-to-hand combat instructors from tactical units around the world, operating in civilian, law enforcement, and military contexts. According to many professionals who have experienced Krav Maga training, the most important and prominent characteristics of the system are the following: (1) The system is comprised of simple, easy-to-learn techniques based on natural body movements and logical defense principles, (2) consequently, practitioners can attain a high level of proficiency in a relatively short period of instruction, (3) the techniques and tactics work even in harsh, uncontrolled and violent environments, (4) individuals retain the ability to perform the techniques at a high level with minimal review and practice.

This publication contains a significant part of the complete system of Krav Maga, including advanced techniques. Our purpose is to intensify the public's awareness of self-defense options as they apply to coping with an **armed aggressor**. The decision to publish this subject matter before other, more fundamental topics in Krav Maga is due, regrettably, to the tide of global violence sweeping most parts of the world in both developed and developing countries. The ever-increasing use of weapons to commit acts of violence against the innocent was the motivating factor behind our selection of subjects for inclusion in this first publication. The next volume will include the fundamentals of self-defense and fighting skills, according to the Krav Maga discipline, against an **unarmed assailant** who may be well-trained or exceedingly powerful, and could present a serious challenge for the defender.

On a professional level, we perceive little difference between a terrorist operation based on nationalistic ideals (for instance, the seizing of an airplane, a ship, or a bus full of passengers), and a situation motivated purely by criminal intent, such as a takeover during the course of a bank robbery, or a kidnapping. In either case, the outcome of the violent encounter will be determined by the correct response at the proper time, and the ability to perform under stress (which could be acquired through Krav Maga training), will enable one to survive unharmed or with minimal injury. Our goal is for the reader to arouse his or her awareness and develop the ability to defend against a violent attack. Clearly, developing such ability leads to greater self-confidence and personal safety, usually resulting in a better quality of life.

Although originally developed for the Israeli Army, Krav Maga has been thoroughly adapted to suit the needs of civilian life as well. Its founder devoted his life to creating a system that **everyone, young and old, man and woman, can use** to defend themselves or their companions when faced with a violent confrontation. This system was carefully designed so that its effectiveness does not depend on one's physical ability. The easy-to-perform, natural techniques, combined with logically structured defense tactics, form a self-defense system characterized by simplicity; this is in fact the true secret of Krav Maga's effectiveness.

In addition to the technical sections of this book that deal with different types of armed attacks, there are important training methods designed to develop the student's ability. Various theoretical subjects are also included to support the training methods, techniques, and tactics. These subjects are aimed at improving one's capacity to perform under stress and minimize the time needed to identify the danger and promptly react to it. The authors direct your attention to Chapter 14: **Safety in Training,** which is entirely devoted to this crucial subject and **must be read thoroughly before commencing any of the physical activities mentioned in this book!**

At the end of the book, we present background material on the history of Krav Maga and its founder, its development over the years, and a chapter about the authors. This is followed by appendices, including information on the editor and the publisher of this book, and a glossary of terms commonly used in Krav Maga.

The authors wish to thank all those who took part in the preparation and publication of this book, and especially Mr. Darren Levine of Los Angeles, California. Mr. Levine, as a technical adviser and professional editor of the book, contributed much of his knowledge and experience in Krav Maga training, as well as his proficiency in the English language. Much of the text appearing in this volume owes its clarity to his voluntary efforts.

The authors and publisher are grateful to the Krav Maga Association of America, Inc., for its ongoing support in the publication of this edition, and to all the talented and devoted individuals who participated in this demanding publishing project and whose persistent efforts have made it possible (see Acknowledgment).

We genuinely hope that you, the reader, will never be in a situation that requires use of the self-defense techniques described herein, but should you encounter such a situation, that you readily apply these techniques without hesitation, confidently and successfully.

Imi Sde-Or and Eyal Yanilov

Netanya, Israel

What is Krav Maga?

Krav Maga, meaning in Hebrew "contact fight", is the official system of self-defense and hand-to-hand combat of the Israel Defense Forces (IDF), the Israeli National Police and other security services. Krav Maga is also taught extensively in public schools and educational centers affiliated with the Israeli Ministry of Education.

Krav Maga was created by the late Imi Sde-Or (Lichtenfeld), who developed the system during his remarkable military career as Chief Instructor of Hand-to-Hand Combat with the IDF. During his service, Imi wrote the army's official self-defense and hand-to-hand combat manual. In 1964 he left the military, though continued to supervise the instruction of Krav Maga in both military and law-enforcement contexts, and in addition, worked indefatigably to refine, improve and adapt Krav Maga to meet civilians needs.

Krav Maga is a modern, practical and proven system of self-defense, carefully conceived for today's volatile world. It is characterized by a logical and coherent approach to self-defense and fighting confrontations that enables one to achieve a relatively high level of proficiency within a short period of instruction. Krav Maga was meticulously developed to be diversified, and thus is applicable to the military, law-enforcement agencies, and civilians alike. The system has consistently earned the praise of experienced fighters, Martial Arts experts, and military and police officers for its highly practical applications, but in essence it also appeals to beginners because of its simple, no-nonsense and realistic approach to personal safety. In fact, Krav Maga is the ideal self-defense method for men, women, young and elderly people of all ages and physical abilities.

In examining the Krav Maga discipline, there are two integral and interrelated components to it: **self-defense** and **hand-to-hand combat** (fighting confrontation).

What is Self-Defense?

After a long day of work, you are walking through the parking lot to your car. Just as you open the door, someone approaches you from behind and puts a knife to your throat. You respond swiftly and aggressively, defending yourself, controlling the weapon and neutralizing the attacker. This is Krav Maga – Self-Defense.

Self-defense is the foundation of the Krav Maga system. Its various techniques have been developed to enable those who train in Krav Maga to defend themselves and others against hostile, violent actions, avoid injury, and overcome and neutralize their assailants. Krav Maga's self-defense techniques include defenses against a wide variety of unarmed though dangerous assaults such as punches, kicks, chokes, head locks, bear hugs, and other holds. They also apply to higher-risk, life-threatening scenarios, where the assailant is armed with a weapon such as a stick, a knife, a gun, or even a hand grenade.

In the early phase of its development, Grandmaster Imi Sde-Or, founder of Krav Maga, was faced with the need to educate efficiently and quickly a wide variety of Israeli soldiers, from physically fit high school graduates to out-of-shape reserve soldiers in their forties. Thus he developed a system that relied on simple, instinctive movements rather than rigid techniques requiring years of training. As a result, the self-defense techniques of Krav Maga can be used effectively by men and women of all different physical characteristics, capabilities, strengths, and ages.

The defensive techniques and principles of Krav Maga are comprised of simple and natural movements that are highly effective and easy to learn. Students are taught to apply these principles and techniques in a variety of situations, from dark surroundings, to a sitting or lying position, or in adverse circumstances where they must defend themselves when their ability to move is severely impeded.

What is Hand-to-Hand Combat?

A man confronts you. He pushes you back with both hands. Until the next move is made, neither of you has an advantage. A flurry of attacks, involving kicks, punches, and the relevant defenses and body movements, is likely to erupt. You are now fully involved in a real fighting confrontation. Hand-to-hand combat constitutes a more sophisticated phase of Krav Maga, where students are taught how to neutralize the adversary quickly and effectively. This part of the system deals with the elements that are related to the actual management of the fight: attacks, defenses, timing, feints, tactics, movements, and vision, along with some important psychological and mental considerations associated with surviving a violent encounter of this type.

Note: Even a strictly self-defense incident where you responded with a specific technique to a certain attack, could easily develop into a full-scale fight. For example, if after following your defense and counterattack, the assailant has not been defeated, and continues to attack, you will find yourself involved in an actual fight.

The Development of Krav Maga

When we try to comprehend the motives behind the development of the Krav Maga discipline, we find them closely related to the background of its founder. (See Chap. 15: **About the Authors**.) In his youth, in Czechoslovakia during the thirties, Grandmaster Imi Sde-Or was well known as a champion athlete in several sports, mainly wrestling and boxing. He was also influenced by his father, who was Chief

Detective and Self-Defense Instructor in the police force and taught Imi several sports and fighting skills, as well as by the many brutal street fights in Bratislava, Imi's home town, that he had to endure (against the National Nazi youth gangs). Furthermore, in dealing with a situation or event that is both violent and dangerous, Imi always applied his natural ability to devise an ingenious technical solution that was very simple yet highly effective.

Krav Maga consists of various physical techniques, though it also instills in the practitioner a unique mental discipline designed to strengthen his (or her) fighting spirit. Special training methods are used to simulate the stress of a real attack, preparing you for the harshness and reality of a true fight for your life. These training methods have been used in Israel's most celebrated elite combat units and have proven themselves in countless actual fighting situations.

The lethal nature of the Krav Maga techniques is perfectly suited to real-life conditions. The system prepares us to cope with our ever-violent world, and enables the practitioner to protect and save lives. It emerged from an environment where violence, mostly of a political nature, was unfortunately commonplace. As a result, Krav Maga is the world's most battle-tested system of self-defense and hand-to-hand combat, having had ample opportunity over the years to be tested, checked and improved.

In recent years, Krav Maga has been taught to civilians and law-enforcement agencies in many different countries throughout the world. It has rapidly gained international recognition from professionals and Martial Arts organizations as a most effective and practical school of self-defense and fighting skills, following the vision of its creator, Grandmaster Imi Sde-Or: "*… that one may walk in peace.*"

The Basic Premises of Krav Maga

As emphasized by its founder, Imi Sde-Or, the basic premises of Krav Maga are:

- **"Do not get hurt"**: Meaning, achieve a high level of proficiency in self-defense. However, if you do get hurt, you must know how to absorb the attack (kick, strike, etc.) and take the correct action under the newly established conditions.

- **"Be modest"**: Do not boast about your skill, and avoid unnecessary conflicts. Overcome your ego and control your mental state, so that they will not fail you during a confrontation. Be ready to accept criticism and instruction from others.

- **"Act correctly"**: Do the right thing at the right place and the right time. Your physical and mental state dictates your ability to handle a confrontation. Make full use of your abilities, and take full advantage of the elements and conditions that prevail in your surroundings, in order to deal effectively with the situation.

• **"Become proficient, so that you will not have to kill"**: The skilled Krav Maga practitioner does not need to inflict unnecessary harm upon his (or her) opponent, and is capable of concluding the confrontation briefly and efficiently. Cultivate consideration for your fellow men, even during a dangerous encounter. On the other hand, heed the ancient expression: *"If someone comes to kill you, kill him first,"* referring to specific situations in which you have no choice, because "it is either him or you."

It is also essential to sharpen one's ability to discern levels of severity of a possible attack. This is especially important for young people, who must be taught the values of self-control and avoiding violence, but who must also acquire the ability to defend themselves effectively. This approach means: first, try to avoid the confrontation, but if you are attacked, **respond with an appropriate degree of strength**, sufficient to neutralize the threat and remove yourself from danger.

Guiding Principles for Krav Maga Techniques

• **Avoid injury**! Carefully calculate the risks involved in a specific action, and avoid danger whenever possible. The basic approach to your actions should be self-defense; **Krav Maga strongly emphasizes the use of defense techniques**.

• The Krav Maga techniques were developed as an extension of the **body's natural reflexes**. These natural responses were then refined, polished and directed to meet the needs of the defender in a given situation.

• Defend and counterattack in the **shortest and most direct way possible**, from any starting position, taking into consideration the safety and convenience of your action.

• **Respond correctly, in accordance with and as required by the circumstances**, carefully checking the nature of your response and the force of the attack (in order to avoid unnecessary injury).

• **Strike correctly at any vulnerable point**, as needed to prevail over the assailant.

• **Use any tool or object available nearby** for your defense and counterattack.

• **In Krav Maga there are no rules**, technical limitations or sportsmanship restrictions.

• The underlying **principle in training**: advancing from closed skill to open skill (incorporating "mental training"), and from a single, specifically defined technique to improvised action in accordance with the dynamics of the situation.

Defense against Knife Attack

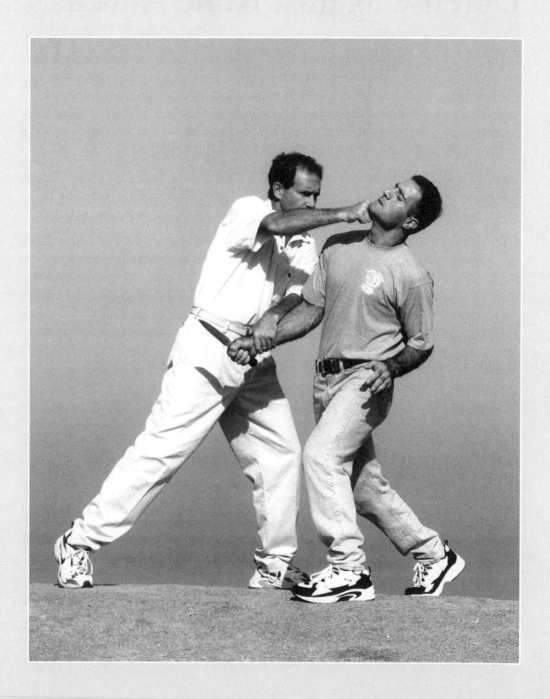

Chapter 1

Defense against Knife Attack

In the Krav Maga system practical defenses were developed to effectively deal with an assailant armed with a sharp-edged weapon. This chapter does not cover the entire subject of knife attacks; it does, however, address defensive principles, tactics, and specific techniques against the most commonly used knife attacks. Scenarios include close, intermediate, and long-range defenses from various angles, as well as disarming and finishing techniques.

This book deals with the subject of facing an assailant armed with a knife, **from the aspect of self-defense**, i.e., when you are **defending** yourself against a knife attack and not as an **active combatant** involved in a fighting confrontation.

Krav Maga places special emphasis on defensive techniques against an assailant armed with a knife and other commonly used sharp-edged objects such as broken bottles, razor blades, scissors, etc. It is necessary to demonstrate and explain the different ways to hold the knife and the various possible attacks. This will enable you to identify the type of attack being delivered among the various stabbing and slashing techniques. Only then will you be able to apply the most effective defense.

Basic Principles of Defense against Knife Attack

- If at all possible, such confrontation should be avoided. Sometimes the best way to do this is simply to flee the scene, especially when you are able to run fast.

- At the moment you notice an assailant coming towards you, with intent to attack, he may be at a number of different **possible ranges**. We differentiate between four main ranges:

  The first: **very close range**, at which you cannot defend yourself unless you are extremely lucky.

  The second: **close range**, where a hand defense will suit. At this range you can defend yourself effectively, particularly against a circular attack.

  The third: **medium range**, where a hand defense together with a suitable body defense can be used to increase the effectiveness of the defense and counterattack, and in order to "catch" the assailant at a relatively early stage.

  The fourth: **long range**, where you can hit the assailant with an intercepting kick and stop him at a relatively long range before he can hurt you.

- Whenever possible, in defending against a knife-wielding assailant **it is important to keep a safe distance**. This will force the would-be stabber to bridge a considerable gap in order to reach his target, giving you the time to take the necessary measures to defend yourself. During this time, you may even be able to find an object nearby and use it to your advantage. Useful objects may include a chair or a stick, with which you can defend yourself or even strike the assailant, or a small rock that can be thrown. (See Chap. 7: **Using Everyday Objects as Defensive Weapons**.)

- If you have enough time, **observe how the attacker is holding the knife**; this will give you some indication as to the type of attacks he is liable to deliver and, accordingly, the possibilities for your defense techniques.

- We must bear in mind that **the human leg is stronger and has greater reach than the arm**. It is therefore preferable in most cases to defend yourself with kicks, and to be at the proper distance in order to execute them. This distance will also serve as the safety margin that will enable you to attack first, before the assailant gets close enough to inflict damage to vital or vulnerable parts of your body.

- When using a hand defense against knife attack, **the counterattack must be executed at top speed**, and it is highly recommended to **grab the hand holding the knife**, so as to keep the attacker from using it again. This is because the typical stabber is generally "programmed" to stab not only once, but **several times**! The defense and the simultaneous counterattack are designed to end the confrontation as soon as possible, so that the attacker will not be able to deliver multiple stabs.

  The force of the impact delivered in the counterattack hampers the attacker's ability to direct additional stabs at the defender. This interference occurs on two fronts: the first refers to the purely physical context, and the second is the effect upon the chain of events that are in motion from the moment the attacker consciously decides to attack and the physiological-neurological events that follow to carry out these attacks.

  In a purely physical context, the strong impact of the defender's counterattack can entirely halt or thwart the attacker's second and subsequent stabs. Even though a second stab is about to be directed at the defender, the defender's strong punch to the attacker's throat or chin will break the attacker's strength, arm speed, weight, momentum, etc.

  In a neurophysical sense, a strong counterattack breaks the chain of events required for the attacker to stab a second or subsequent times. In effect, the impact of the counterattack to the head may interrupt the brain transmission instructing the assailant's body to attack in multiple sequence: it "jams" the necessary signals that would have resulted in the subsequent attack (or attacks).

- **Appropriate body defenses** should be included in the various defensive techniques for evading the attack. This will serve as an additional safety factor in case the hand defense was not completely successful, and will also minimize the possibility of your being cut by a second attack.

- A stab (or any other attack) is stronger and more dangerous if the attacking limb covered a considerable distance and accumulated speed and power. Therefore, we should strive to execute the defense and thwart the attack **before** the hand holding the knife has had time to gain full momentum, i.e., when it is still close to the attacker's body.

- Although Krav Maga clearly favors **combining the defense and counterattack simultaneously**, there are situations where this may be difficult to accomplish, e.g., when the attack is sudden and unexpected. Under these circumstances, you may only be able to respond with a defense. It is therefore extremely important to regain your composure immediately and **counterattack forcefully at the first opportunity**, and as soon as possible neutralize (and control) the hand that is holding the knife. **Remember**: Even though the defense prevents the initial attack, it is mainly your counterattack that saves lives and prevents the assailant from achieving his (or her) objective.

- If possible, when using hand defense techniques, **advance towards the attacker**. This will place you in the proper range to execute the counterattacks, enabling you to overcome the assailant and prevent him from changing his angle of approach in order to stab again.

- If you noticed the approaching knife attack at the last moment, **a quick leap in the right direction**, with or without a hand defense, may put you out of range. From your new position, you will find it easier to defend and attack at angles more convenient to you.

- **The incident is over** when you succeed in removing yourself from the scene of danger or when the assailant cannot or does not want to attack again (because he has given up, been knocked out, fled the scene, etc.) If you remain at the scene you should disarm the adversary, either by taking his knife or tossing it away, so that it may not be used again by the assailant or any third party.

- **You will probably be surprised by the attack**. An assailant armed with a knife or other sharp-edged weapon will often conceal the fact that he is carrying a weapon. In fact, victims who have survived a violent confrontation against a knife-wielding assailant consistently report that they were completely unaware of the existence of the weapon until after they had suffered stab or slash wounds. In essence, these survivors of edged weapon attacks state that they believed they were engaged in some sort of fist fight; only later, after sustaining injuries, did they realize that the assailant was armed with a cutting instrument. Simply stated, one may not initially see the knife at the early stages of a fight. First of all, one should learn to pay some attention to the assailant's hands: look to see if, in fact, he is armed. Secondly, when considering the question of how we should ideally stand when facing an assailant armed with a knife, we must consider at what stage it was, when we became aware of the edged weapon.

- **Your initial stance**
  If you notice at the very onset of the confrontation that the assailant is armed with a knife, **remain in a neutral or passive stance**. Perform the defensive technique from this position. Being ready, although assuming a position close to a passive or neutral stance, will possibly encourage the assailant to attack in a straightforward manner without creating deception or using other tactics with his attack, thereby making it more difficult to defend.

  However, if you become aware of the knife while the fight is already in progress, do not switch back to a passive or neutral position. Your stance should first "invite" the attack to a specific opening, to the location which you are ready to defend, and then be organized so that your arms, hands, and fingers are brought in closer to your body and will not be cut or slashed.

Training Hints

- When training with a partner, a soft knife (made of rubber, for example) should be used for the initial exercises, until the student has become skilled enough in defending himself against high-speed, high-power attacks. Only then may he begin training with a harder knife, e.g., made of wood or plastic. **A sharp metal knife may be used only in the advanced stages of training, observing all required safety measures**. The student, while still in the learning phase, must become accustomed to the feel of defending himself against an attack with a real knife.

- It is recommended that during the initial stages of training, the partner playing the role of assailant **wear a forearm guard on the arm holding the knife**. This will allow him to attack with the required speed and force, without fear of pain or injury from the defenses that will be applied against his forearm.

A Real-Life Story

A novice student in kick-boxing from Finland, underwent basic training in Krav Maga in defense against assailants armed with a knife. Shortly afterwards, he was attacked in a nightclub and the assailant attempted to stab him in the neck. The student performed the defense technique that he had learned, and at the same time counter-attacked with a punch to the chin. The attacker fell and lost consciousness.

Holding the Knife

Regular or "Ice Pick" Hold

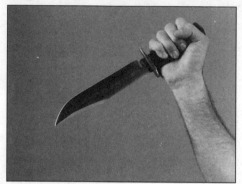

Holding the knife

The Bowie knife has an asymmetric blade, usually sharpened on one side only. With this type of knife, the point of the blade shall face downward, as shown in the photograph, in order to facilitate penetration.

The stab: Executed vertically from top to bottom, or diagonally inward. For common stabbing method: see aggressor in the techniques for defending against this type of stab.

Oriental Hold

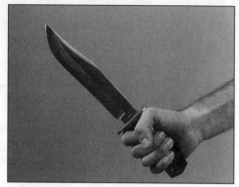

Holding the knife

When one is using a Bowie knife, as described above, the point shall face upward, as shown in the photograph.

The stab: Executed vertically upward or diagonally inward. For common stabbing method, see aggressor in the various defense techniques against this type of stab.

Straight Hold

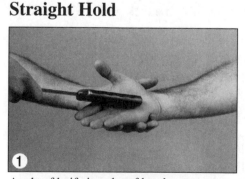

① Angle of knife in palm of hand

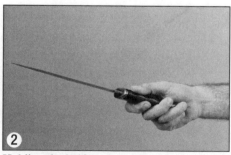

② Holding the knife

The hold: Position the knife diagonally in the palm of your hand. In order for the blade to be horizontal during the stab, it must be held at an angle of approximately 45° relative to the palm surface. To prevent the knife from slipping backward during the stab, place the base of the handle against the heel of your hand, with the thumb pressing on the middle of the handle. This will make it possible to deliver a strong and steady straight stab.

The stab: Done with a straight movement, similar to a punch; the foot parallel to the stabbing hand is usually in front. Common stabbing method: see aggressor in the defense techniques against this type of stab.

Slash Hold

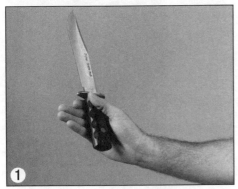

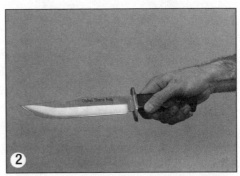

①
Grip on knife before slashing

②
Grip on knife while slashing horizontally (taken from above)

The hold: The knife angle and blade position relative to the palm of the hand are similar to those in the **straight hold**, but this time you could move the handle in the palm of your hand. In this case the axis of movement is between the thumb and index finger, and the knife handle is not pressed against the heel of the hand. The thumb is slightly to the side of the handle, with the lower inside part of the thumb pressing the knife into the palm of the hand.

The slash: Executed by moving the hand from side to side, either horizontally or diagonally. While slashing from the outside to the inside, the fingers clasp the knife handle inside the palm of your hand, adding to the speed of the knife at the moment of impact and also increasing the strength of the hold.

A slash to the outside can be delivered in two ways, depending upon whether the knife has a single or double-edged blade. If the knife has a single-edged blade (like the Bowie knife, for example), the forearm should rotate so that the single-edged blade and the palm of the hand face outward into the direction of the slash. If the knife has a double-edged blade, no rotation is necessary; the back of the hand simply moves out toward the target. Another consideration favoring rotation of the knife (so that the palm of the hand leads to the target) is the fact that the knife itself is more secure in the hand upon impact.

Note: One can perform a slashing attack with a knife held in other ways too!

Defenses against Downward Stab: Knife in Regular ("Ice Pick") Hold

Sudden Stab from the Front – Regular Hold

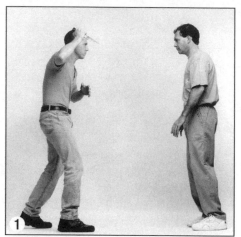

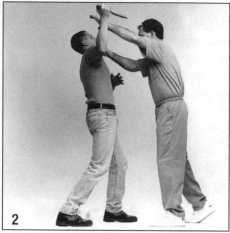

The aggressor is positioned in front of you, a short distance away, and suddenly delivers an "ice pick" stab from the front. He may need to take a short step in order to reach you.

Execute a forearm defense, thrusting your shoulder in the direction of the defense, and counterattacking simultaneously with a straight punch to the assailant's chin or neck. (Under less surprising circumstances, it is recommended also to advance with a short step.)

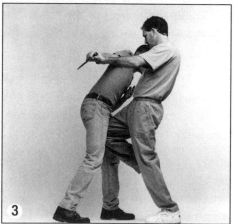

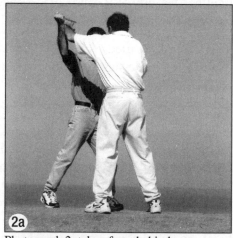

With your defending arm, push and grab the hand holding the knife with the palm of your hand or with a "hook-like" handhold and apply continuous pressure against it, which will hinder the attacker's ability to stab again. As early as possible, advance forward, grab the assailant's shoulder or shirt and deliver a knee to his groin.

Photograph 2, taken from behind.

The hard (bony) part of your forearm, approximately midway between the elbow and the tip of the little finger, stops the aggressor's forearm. The forearm defense strikes near the wrist of the stabbing hand. If you notice the attack in time, you can execute the counterattack **simultaneously with the defense**. Time and distance permitting, you will be defending and counterattacking while advancing forward. Under conditions constituting more of a surprise, you may defend first and counterattack immediately thereafter.

As you maintain your hand defense, it is also recommended to advance forward aggressively while counterattacking and applying firm pressure with your forearm, forward and slightly downward on the assailant's forearm, in order to prevent any further use of the knife. It is essential to **grab the attacking forearm** in order to prevent the assailant from pulling his hand back and using the knife again. Do this by pushing and grabbing the assailant's forearm in the palm of your hand, or by hooking your palm around his forearm. This makes it difficult for him to use the knife again, and usually is all that is necessary to **prevent a second stab**, since you are counterattacking throughout this time. At the end of this stage, you should maintain a firm grasp on the assailant's forearm. Finish the encounter by disarming the assailant or by distancing yourself from the danger as early as possible.

Variation: *An important variation of this technique is to execute the hand defense and counterattack (without grabbing the assailant's forearm); continue with a kick to the groin, and then **leave the scene** in a controlled manner.*

Sudden Stab from the Side – Regular Hold

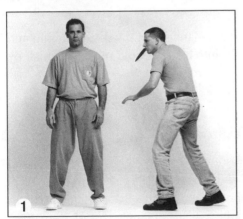

The assailant is almost within stabbing range, and relative to yourself, he is positioned on the side opposite his stabbing hand. Here, for example, the stab is executed with the right hand, with the attacker at your left.

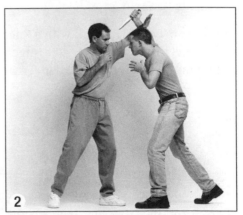

The assailant advances and tries to stab. Noticing this, send your forearm to stop the aggressor's forearm. (While executing the defense, you should also lower your head slightly, between your shoulders.)

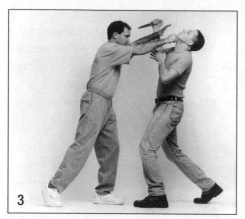

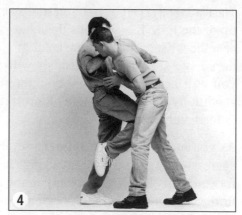

As early as possible, move away quickly or start your counterattack, turning your body and, if necessary, stepping towards the assailant. Apply continuous pressure against the forearm of his stabbing hand, and as early as possible, grab it with the palm of your hand or by hooking your palm around it.

Grab the aggressor's clothing or his shoulder, grasping forcefully with your fingers. Finish with a knee to his groin.

This technique can be executed more effectively **if you observe the oncoming attack in time**, since it is then possible to defend, turn, and counterattack simultaneously. Defense against a more sudden and surprising stab is executed as a single action: your forearm blocks the aggressor's forearm. In a continuous movement, execute a counterattack, simultaneously applying pressure against the attacking forearm and grabbing it firmly to prevent the attacker from pulling back his hand and stabbing again.

Continue the counterattack with a knee to the assailant's groin, while grabbing and pulling his shirt or digging your fingers deeply into his trapezoid muscle. Finish by distancing yourself from the danger zone.

A Real-Life Story

David entered the elevator on the ground floor of a residential building in New York. The elevator stopped at one of the lower floors and another man got in, who looked and acted suspiciously. Seconds after the elevator began moving again, the man put his hand inside the pocket of his jacket. David, sensing possible danger, grabbed the man's forearm and struck him. When he pulled the man's hand out of the pocket, it was holding a large switchblade knife.

Sudden Stab from the "Live" Side – Regular Hold

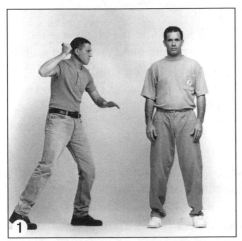

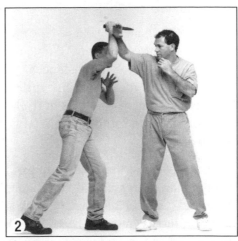

The assailant is almost within stabbing range and, relative to you, is on the same side as the stabbing hand. Here, for example, the stab is executed with the right hand, while the attacker is on your right.

As the aggressor advances and stabs, execute a forearm defense against his forearm. Continue by moving away quickly, or counterattack as described hereafter.

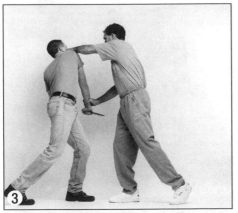

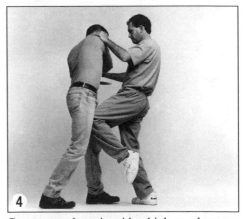

Proceed by pressing against the assailant's forearm, redirecting the stabbing hand by continuously applying sideways and then downward pressure against it, and then grab and secure it. At the same time, deliver a straight or roundhouse punch.

Counterattack again with a kick or a knee to the assailant's groin.

The stab comes from the side, to the area between your upper chest and your neck. The outside defense, with the forearm, is performed as a single, flowing action; it is followed by the counterattack, which is executed at the same time as you are redirecting the assailant's forearm, applying pressure, while grabbing it and bringing it down. If you observe the approaching attack in time, you can **continue the momentum** of the aggressor's attack with a continuous arc-like movement instead of completely stopping the attacking hand at an opposing 90° angle.

On the other hand, if your reaction was slightly delayed and the attacker attempts to stab again, you may not be able to redirect the attacking hand down and grab it. Depending on the circumstances, you may proceed with the following options: Turn towards the assailant while defending with your rear (left) hand and counterattacking with the front (right) hand; jump away from the attacker; defend yourself and control the additional stab; deliver a side kick to the assailant's knee or lower ribs.

Note: These last three techniques, depicted here for defense against a sudden, regular stab, are essentially the same. You execute a basic forearm defense to stop the attack, and send a counterattack as early and as fast as possible to a vulnerable point on the aggressor's head. You then continue as needed: counterattack again, disarm the opponent, leave the scene, etc.

Stab, Regular Hold – Kick to the Groin

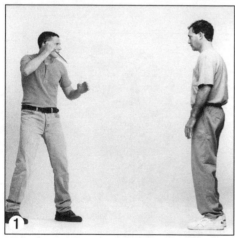

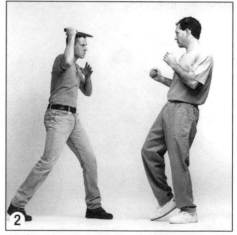

You observe the approaching attack when the assailant is two or three steps away from stabbing distance.

At the same time as the assailant is moving forward and preparing to stab, advance with a quick, diagonal forward stomping step and send the kicking leg towards the center of the assailant's body.

The nature of the stab is a powerful strike directed diagonally downward and inward (along a line from above and beside the assailant's shoulder, down to his opposite hip). This is preceded by an advance, in which the assailant is slightly bending his upper body backwards to achieve a powerful attack; this causes him to expose his groin area.

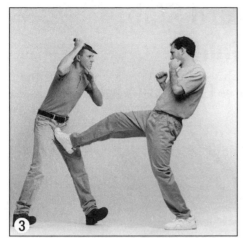

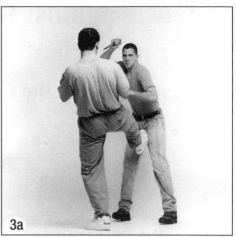

Deliver a regular kick to the groin, to stop the assailant and neutralize him at a safe distance. Strike with the ball of your foot. The assailant is hit while moving forward and his arm is thrown backwards, long before he lands his attack. Thrust the hip of the kicking leg forward to achieve maximum range and power.

Photograph 3, taken from behind: Attack with a swift kick to the groin, directed upward and forward (striking with the ball of the foot) to stop the assailant before he sends his stabbing hand towards you.

The attack is a regular kick to the groin, hitting with the ball of the foot. Execute it while thrusting the hip of the kicking leg forward, in order to achieve maximum reach and power. The angle of attack to the groin is roughly 45° diagonally upward and forward; the kick stops the assailant **while he is still relatively far away and cannot reach you with his knife**, since his arm is thrown backward.

While the assailant advances and prepares to stab, you are advancing and kicking. The type of advance depends on how far away the attacker is and on your intentions, as explained below.

Option 1: As depicted here, advance with a quick stomping step diagonally forward and out, to remove yourself from the line of attack. This brings the kicking (right) leg forward to the center of the target, and keeps it from colliding with the forward leg of the assailant.

Option 2: Without advancing, stomp lightly in place with one foot (the left); this foot now bears your weight. With the other foot, kick the assailant in the groin, while executing a slight body turn. This option is useful when the initial distance between you and the assailant is relatively short (or if you prefer to wait until the aggressor is within kicking range).

Variation: If you prefer to kick with your left, advance diagonally forward and to the right on your right leg and kick with your left; avoid hitting the assailant's legs.

Defenses against Upward Stab: Knife in "Oriental" Hold

Sudden Stab from the Front – Oriental Hold

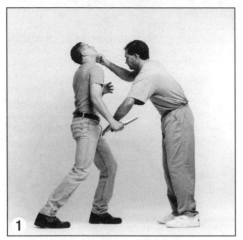

1

The aggressor surprises you at close range. Lean forward, execute a forearm defense accompanied by a counterattack: a straight punch to the face. If possible, perform the defense and counterattack **simultaneously**.

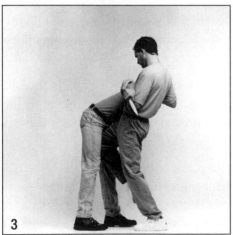

3

Grab the assailant's forearm and knee him in the groin. On how to trap his forearm, see *Threat from Behind, at Close Range* in Chap. 4: **Neutralizing a Threat at Gunpoint**.

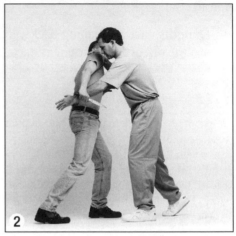

2

If you chose to continue with control and counterattacks, advance forward and push against the attacker's forearm, turning your palm (with thumb facing out) and sending it forward and out. Grab the assailant's shoulder or trapezoid muscle in order to control him more effectively.

The attack described here is sudden, frontal, and at short range. The defending forearm is the one opposite the attacking forearm. It stops the attack with the elbow bent, meeting the assailant's forearm near the wrist. Your upper body leans forward, keeping the knife from reaching your stomach. It is very important to keep your knees straight and not bent; this enables you to maintain a greater distance between yourself and the knife. Along with the defense, execute an attack: a straight punch to the face or throat of the assailant.

In order to execute the defense and counterattack simultaneously, **the approaching attack must have been observed in time**. Otherwise, you will need to execute the counterattack immediately after the defense, since when taken by surprise it is difficult to perform two different kind of movements at the same time, i.e., defense and counterattack.

You have a number of options for further action after executing your defense and initial counterattack:

- Gain distance by leaping backwards. This allows you to improve your position, see the effect of the counterattack, and hinder any further development.

- Execute a regular kick to the groin plus additional counterattacks, making sure that your defending hand continues to do its job.

- Advance powerfully forward. As shown here, wrap your arm under and around the attacker's forearm, trapping it forcefully between your upper arm, forearm, chest, and hand, and counterattack (grab as is done against a *Threat from Behind, at Close Range* in Chap. 4: **Neutralizing a Threat at Gunpoint**.)

- If the assailant continues to apply very strong, upward pressure with his forearm against yours, move diagonally forward and grab his wrist. Then, execute the "cavalier" leverage, as in the technique *Stab, Oriental Hold – Diagonal Forearm Defense* (the next technique to be explained in this chapter).

- The decision on how to proceed also depends upon how the counterattack has affected the assailant and how you feel during the incident.

  Remember: There is another recommended option: **simply flee the scene as fast as you can** (especially if you are quick and agile). It might be less heroic but sometimes proves to be much safer!

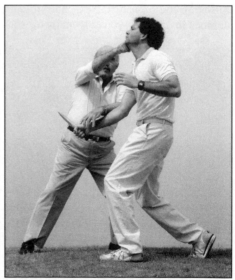

Grandmaster Imi demonstrating a defense technique against knife attack in Oriental hold.

Stab, Oriental Hold – Diagonal Forearm Defense

This defense is executed when you are fortunate enough to see the attacker in advance, but he is too close for you to kick him. This technique is also suitable if you do not feel comfortable or confident with high kicks; or, perhaps, if you simply prefer this defense.

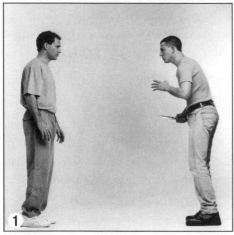

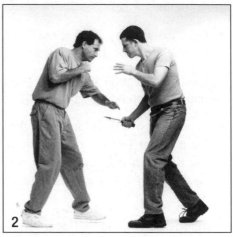

The assailant, armed with a knife, prepares to stab you.

Photograph 2: The assailant advances, intending to stab. Burst forward and execute a forearm defense that "pulls" you diagonally forward, with your upper body leaning forward as well. This is accompanied by a quick turn of your body, which essentially removes you from the line of danger. This part of the defense is referred to as an evasion technique or "body defense."

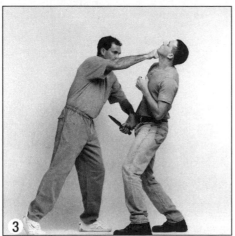

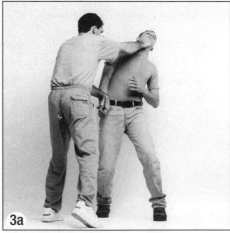

Execute a forearm defense and a body turn; grab the attacker's forearm or wrist and punch him in the chin, all at the same time and shifting your weight forward.

Photograph 3, taken from behind: Continue by removing yourself from the danger zone, or proceed as described in photograph 4 and subsequently.

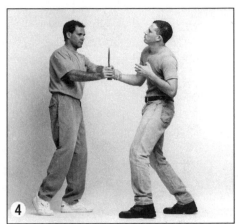

4

With a secure grip, grab the attacker's hand that is holding the knife, and distance yourself from the danger zone of the knife and the assailant, changing the position of your feet.

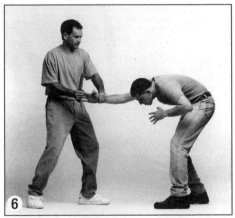

6

Bend the assailant's wrist and dig your fingers forcefully into the palm of the hand holding the knife, alongside the handle, and with a scraping movement remove the knife from the assailant's hand.

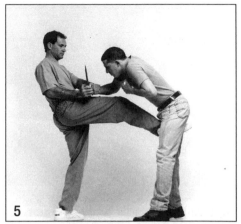

5

Deliver a regular kick to the attacker's groin. This may be followed, by taking the knife, as explained in photograph 6.

In an optimal defense, all the moves described in photographs 2 and 3 **are executed simultaneously and in one flowing movement**. However, during the learning stage, this phase should be divided into two parts:
(1) Forearm defense with forward lunge accompanied by body turn.
(2) Grabbing the aggressor's forearm and counterattacking.

Caution: In Oriental holds, there is always the danger that the assailant will stab **diagonally and almost horizontally inward**, rather than upward. Therefore, it is preferable, in most cases, to deliver a kick to the assailant's chin, similar to the defense against attacks from long range. This will be explained later in the chapter. Therefore, when you decide to use this technique, in order to be protected from the danger mentioned above, you must act as follows: Burst diagonally forward and meet the aggressor's forearm with your defending forearm, as close as possible to the assailant's body, to prevent the stabbing arm from advancing in unexpected directions and before the attack gains considerable momentum, strength, and speed. The position of the defending forearm offers a good defense even against the diagonal stab, almost without moving your elbow, or at most, moving it only an inch or two.

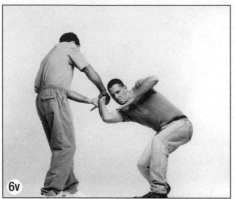

An example of another possibility: drop the aggressor to the ground by applying leverage to his wrist (the "cavalier" leverage).

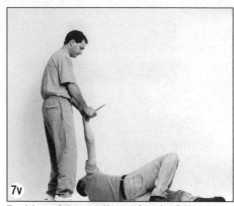

Position of the assailant, after the fall.

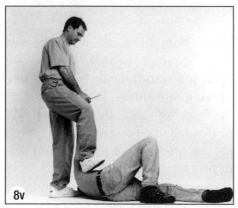

If necessary, kick the assailant in the ribs or kidney and then take the knife from his hand, as described in photograph 6.

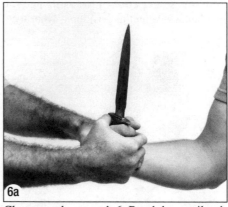

Close-up, photograph 6: Bend the assailant's wrist.

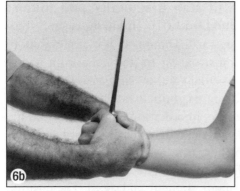

Close-up, photograph 6: Dig your fingers into the assailant's palm.

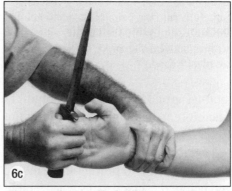

Close-up, photograph 6: With a scraping movement, grab the knife handle and remove the knife from the assailant's hand.

Remember: **Body movement is an important element of the defense**. Its purpose is to remove yourself from the line of attack, by advancing diagonally forward and turning your body. The counterattack, a straight punch to the chin or throat, must be executed as early as possible, and sometimes can be done even before the forearm defense has met the attack. This is an especially powerful counterattack due to the position of your body (leaning forward) and the fact that the punch is delivered to the aggressor's body as he moves towards you to complete his attack.

The entire incident may be over quite rapidly, possibly even right after the first counterattack. It is hoped that the counterattack will succeed in causing the assailant to fall or drop his knife; if not, kick him in the groin and execute additional counterattacks. You may also use the **cavalier leverage**, a technique applied to the wrist of the hand holding the knife, twisting the wrist while bending it outward and pressing down on the back of the hand, causing the assailant to fall to the ground. This leverage is discussed in detail in the section **Neutralizing a Threat of Hand Grenade** (in Chap. 6: **Hostage Situations**).

Once the aggressor has fallen, you can execute additional counterattacks such as kicks to the kidney area or, in certain situations, stomping kicks to his head.

Caution: These counterattacks are liable to be fatal, and therefore **shall not be used unless your life is still in danger** after the assailant has been knocked to the ground by the counterattack!

Note: Using the cavalier leverage and disarming the attacker, as explained here, are intended mainly for police officers and others who prefer not to attack with anything stronger than a punch (for instance, against a teenager holding a knife). In other words, after the defense and the punch, the aggressor is brought down by the relatively gentle cavalier technique, and the knife is removed from his hand.

There are three basic options for taking the knife from the hand of the attacker: (1) "**Scraping**" it from his hand, whether or not he is lying down. (2) **Punching** the back of his hand so that the knife is thrown aside. (3) **Applying a leverage action** to the assailant's wrist, once he has been thrown down on his back, with the elbow of the arm holding the knife pressed against the ground. The pressure loosens the attacker's grip on the knife, and the knife falls from his hand to your hand or to the ground. Strong pressure may even break his wrist.

Note: If you use one hand to pick up the knife from the ground, you must keep the other ready for attack or defense!

Stab to the Stomach from the Side, Oriental Hold – Forearm Defense

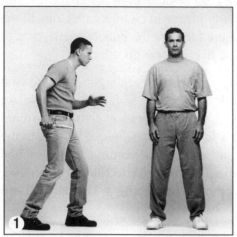

The assailant comes from the same side as his attacking hand or diagonally from that side (in the example shown, he comes from your right side, holding the knife in his right hand).

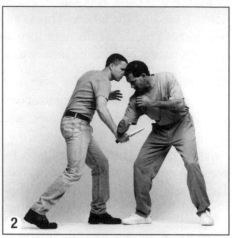

The attacker executes a diagonal stab towards your stomach. Respond with a forearm defense, with your upper body bent. When possible, respond simultaneously with a step diagonally backwards and towards the opponent.

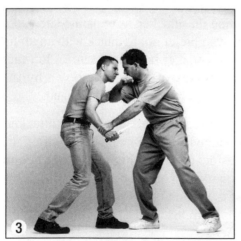

Your defending hand bounces from the defense to a decisive counterattack (consisting of a sideways chop or hammer punch to the attacker's chin, throat, or neck). Simultaneously, you switch hands and grab the assailant's forearm with your other hand.

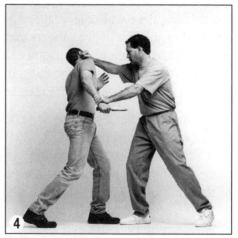

Strike the assailant with a sideways chop or a hammer punch.

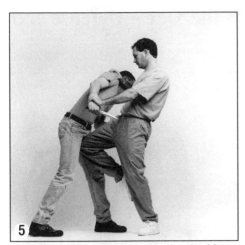

Continue by grabbing the assailant's shirt or shoulder, and knee him with your rear leg; or (as shown) advance with your rear leg in a quick step, kneeing him in the groin with your forward leg.

This technique is appropriate when the assailant prepares to stab you in your ribs or stomach, and you notice the attack in time; move diagonally backwards and towards the assailant while executing the forearm defense.

The defense, which blocks the stab, is performed with a sharp strike that stops the attacker's forearm near the wrist and then "bounces" off his forearm to execute the counterattack. The change of hands is accomplished quickly: the hand in the rear moves forward to grab the assailant's forearm in order to keep him from using the knife again, and the hand that had been defending moves forcefully to execute a chop or lateral hammer punch.

Note: To better prevent any possible reuse of the weapon, when you grab the assailant's hand, push it down and towards him.

Variation: If the attack took you by surprise, or if it is directed towards your ribs or back, then after executing the forearm defense only, you should jump away, distancing yourself from the opponent. This will put you in a better position to continue, rather than remaining close to the assailant and counterattacking. (See the next technique.)

Note: Against an assailant coming from the same angle and side but **stabbing with his left hand** towards your ribs, execute a forearm defense that will deflect or stop the attack. Immediately afterwards, jump aside in order to increase the distance and give yourself the opportunity to operate in the most tactically correct way. This is necessary as the defense creates a situation that makes it difficult to counterattack while preventing the assailant from stabbing again. You should also take this action against an aggressor attacking from your left and holding the knife in his right hand.

Stab to Stomach or Ribs from the Side – Defense and Fast Retreat

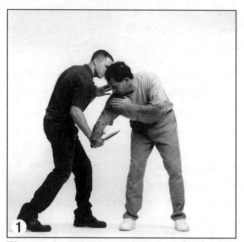 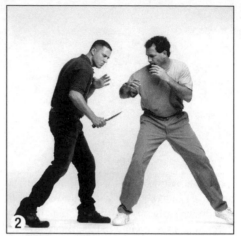

The attacker surprises you from the side with a stab directed at your stomach or ribs. Bend at the waist and block the stab with your forearm at or near his wrist.

Jump away from the assailant, creating a "safety distance" between the two of you. This move will better enable you to respond should he try to launch another attack.

Obviously, when you are surprised, it is difficult to perform any movement other than the reflexive defense. When you find it hard to counterattack and control the hand holding the weapon, you should immediately, as you have no better alternative, distance yourself quickly from the danger zone.

Stab, Oriental Hold – Kick to the Chin

Against this type of attack, it is preferable to use a high, regular (front) kick that **does not pass near the knife**. To hit the assailant's chin effectively (and not in the stomach or chest), you should raise the knee of your kicking leg high, before straightening the leg and kicking. Hit with the ball of your foot.

Body defense: Move out of the line of attack, turning and moving aside, switching the position of your heels with an "exploding" step.

The aggressor is struck by the kick during his advance, his attacking arm is thrown backwards and he is still too far away to reach you with his knife. Based on the timing and the distance from the assailant, you can also **adjust the distance** by retreating or advancing as necessary with a kind of leg-crossing or stomping step.

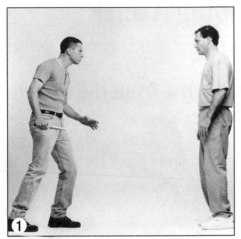

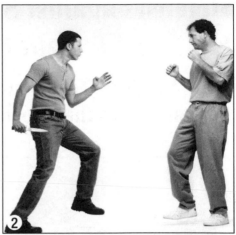

The distance between you and the assailant, once you notice that he is preparing to stab, is relatively long and sufficient for a kick.

The assailant advances. During this time, if you intend to kick him with your right leg, switch the position of your heels with a quick stomping step, turning your body so that the toes of the base (left) foot are directed diagonally outward, thus forming a body defense.

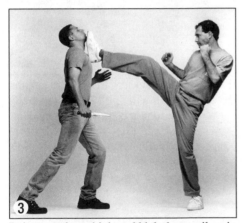

Raise your knee high and kick the assailant in the chin. The hip of your kicking leg is thrust forward to achieve maximum reach and power.

Additional options:

- If time is lacking, you can still kick the stabber's chin from where you are standing, turning your base foot and hip but without the initial movement of changing the position of your heels.

- If you prefer to kick with your other (left) leg, the one directly opposite the attacking (right) hand, advance with your base (right) foot in a stomping step diagonally forward and to the right. This will move you out of the line of attack and minimize the likelihood of your kicking leg being injured by the knife.

Defenses against Stabbing Attack: Knife in Straight Hold

Stab, Straight Hold – Inside Defense from the Outside (Advancing to the "Dead" Side)

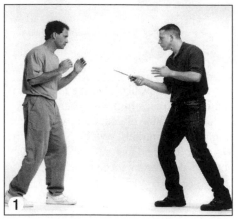

1

When at a safe distance from the aggressor, you are ready for a hand defense. (See note on starting stance.)

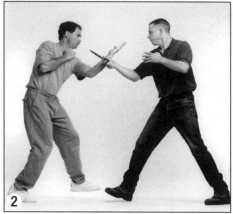

2

The assailant attacks. Start with the forearm defense, which will "pull" you diagonally forward and lead your body defense. The elbow must be low in order to create a greater defensive range and to defend against a possible low stab. At the start of the deflection, your defending forearm comes in contact with the back of the attacker's hand holding the knife.

The forearm defense "leads" your body defense and advance. In this action, send your forearm away from your body, but as perpendicular to the ground as possible. This extends the range of the defense and increases the protected area of your body, which is from the head to the lower abdomen.

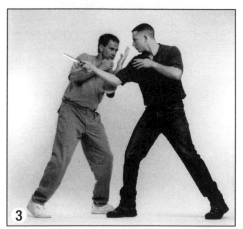

3

The stabbing hand was deflected sideways. The defending forearm slides forward, starting from the wrist or the area in back of the hand, pressing slightly on the attacking forearm up to the area near the assailant's elbow.

The body defense is also important, and both defenses (hand and body) must be executed at top speed!

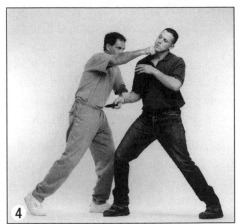

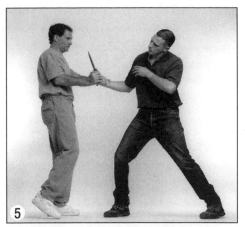

Grab the forearm of the hand holding the knife while executing a powerful counterattack. Depending on whether or not the assailant quickly retracts his hand from the attack, you will grab his arm near the wrist, or possibly even his upper arm near the elbow.

With both hands, hold the attacker's wrist and fist for the "cavalier" leverage, switch legs, and distance yourself from the assailant.

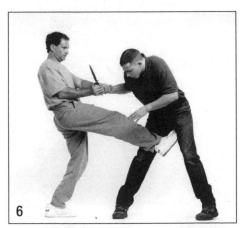

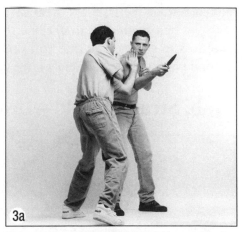

Photograph 3, taken from behind: For an effective defense, the elbow must be low.

Deliver a regular kick to the groin. Take further action as necessary. For example, taking the knife from the assailant, or executing the "cavalier" leverage on the assailant's hand and throwing him to the ground, as previously explained in the section **Defenses against Upward Stab: Knife in "Oriental" Hold**.

Remember that the forearm defense has to be applied at the earliest possible moment, and against the back of the attacker's hand or wrist, **not his forearm**.

Since the aggressor is likely to stab quickly and retract his arm like a spring in order to stab again, it is essential to restrict the movement of the attacking arm. However, **under no circumstances should you grab the knife** when it is brought back. Therefore, you must move your defending arm forward, sliding your forearm along the assailant's to create a "connection" between your forearm and his. The hand of your defending arm will be able to grab the assailant's stabbing arm due to the connection formed. This "connection" will prevent the knife from being redirected at you and allow you to grab the assailant's stabbing arm. If the stab is lower, or if the aggressor is in a low starting stance, you must lower your stance as well so that you can cover the area of your lower abdomen with a forearm defense.

Note: The requirement that you be in the starting stance before applying the technique **pertains to the learning stage only**. Remember that in a real incident, you might have to start from a passive and more neutral stance. Another aspect to consider is that the assailant may try to stab or slash your forward (outstretched) hand if your stance and position "invite" such an action. Therefore, in later practice, before executing the defense, make sure that your hands are close to your body and that the proper foot is slightly forward. This will simulate a less ready position, as might be the case under realistic circumstances (or in a situation in which you do not encourage the assailant to do anything else but execute the most simple, direct stab). When beginning to execute this technique, perform your hand and body defenses in such a way that you simulate the positions depicted in the first and second photographs. Remember, the defending hand leads your movement.

Stab, Straight Hold – Inside Defense to the "Live" Side

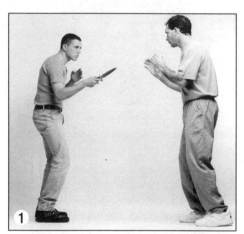

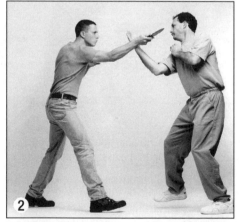

When at a safe distance from the assailant, you are ready to execute a hand defense (see note on starting stance). You will defend with your forward hand (much like the previous technique), but to the inside of the attacker's arm.

The defending forearm, which is thrust forward and almost perpendicular to the ground, strikes the inside of the attacking palm or wrist and deflects it in a sweeping motion, remaining in contact with it for some distance and time.

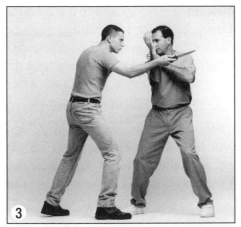

3

Your hand defense is a sweeping motion that redirects the stab. Your forearm defense leads the body defense and diagonal advance forward. As an additional precaution, the body defense involves tilting your body slightly back while the hand defense is performed.

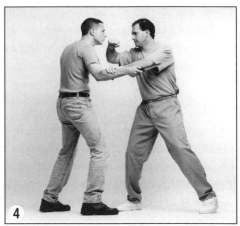

4

Raise the elbow of the defending arm to deliver an effective counterattack. Simultaneously, your rear (left) hand grabs the attacking arm, taking into account its spring-like retreat.

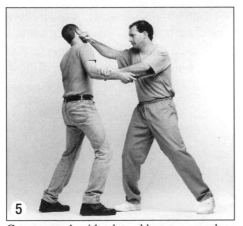

5

Counterattack with a lateral hammer punch or an outward chop to the assailant's head, neck, or throat.

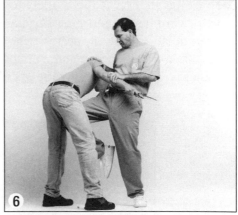

6

Continue by grabbing the assailant's shoulder and delivering a knee to his groin. This can be done with your forward (right) leg after a quick advance with your rear (left) leg, or, as dictated by the angle, you can kick with your rear leg.

Apply the forearm defense near the palm or wrist of the attacking hand. A sweep defense redirects the line of attack. It is needed because of the angle of attack and to avoid the elbow crook. During the defense, keep your other hand close to your neck. Execute the first counterattack (chop or horizontal hammer punch) as early as possible. When delivering your first counterattack, you also send your other hand to grab the assailant's hand.

Caution: A skilled stabber might stab **and then retract his arm like a spring, in order to stab again**! Keep this in mind when sending your rear hand to grab the assailant's. Plan to grab him in the elbow area, so that if the stabbing hand comes back, you will catch it near the wrist. When grabbing the attacker's arm, hold the elbow of your grabbing arm low and apply pressure. This will prevent the knife from being redirected at you with an inward slash-type attack, or another stab.

The body defense is more important when defending with an inside defense to the attacker's live side than it is when defending with an inside defense from the outside (dead side) against the same type of stab. To enhance your body defense, bend back the area that the attacker is aiming at, i.e., if the stab is aimed at your neck, **your upper body should be tilted back**.

Note: Here too, the requirement that the technique be applied from a starting stance, as shown, applies to the learning stage only. In normal, everyday life we do not operate from a fighting stance, and in a true, life-threatening situation we may not have enough time to get into the stance before we perform the technique. Also, in a tactical sense, we may wish to avoid an obvious "defensive" stance so as not to draw the aggressor's attention to the impending defense. We seem to "invite" the stab so the attacker is more likely to deliver a simple, direct stab without slashing our forward hand, feinting, or trying to trick us. Therefore, in order to simulate a more realistic situation, perform the technique from a stance that does not reveal your intent to take action and will not create a psychological threat to the assailant. In other words: **do not show the assailant that you are trained to foil his attacks**.

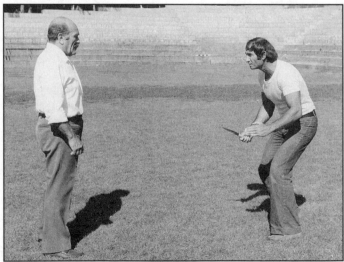

Grandmaster Imi before demonstrating a defense technique against knife attack in Oriental hold.

Sudden Straight Stab Aimed at Lower Abdomen

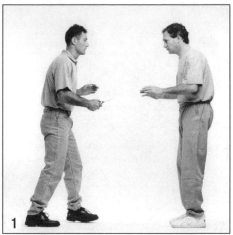

1

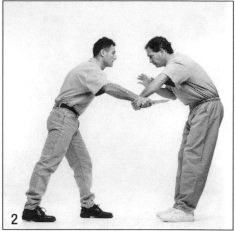

2

The assailant attacks with a straight stab aimed at your lower abdomen. A natural reflexive reaction is to send both hands forward against the stabbing, and to move the pelvis backwards.

Transform this natural hand reaction to an outside scooping defense with your wrist area, sweeping the attack sideways with a small circular movement. Move your pelvis backwards.

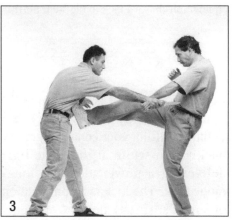

3

Come back quickly with your pelvis, while delivering a forceful kick to the assailant's groin, solar plexus, or chin.

The natural reaction to this "low-altitude" attack, especially if it comes as a surprise, is to distance the pelvis while sending the hands forward.

The hand defense used is a scooping movement with the wrist area. The counterattack will be done towards the end of the hand defense, while quickly returning the pelvis to its previous position and delivering a regular kick to a vulnerable point on the assailant's body. A kick to the solar plexus will also serve to push the assailant back. A competent trainee may be able to deliver a hand strike simultaneously with the hand defense.

*Variations: Other reflexive moves that can be made against this stab are inside defense with an open palm (similar to the one used in the technique **Long-distance Threat from the Front** in the next chapter, **Defense against Impending Threat with a Knife**); or an inside defense with forearm turned, palm down, and elbow up.*

Stab, Straight Hold – Kick to Center of the Body

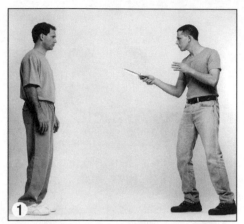

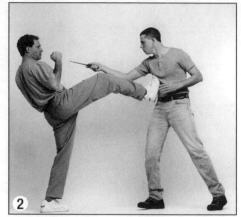

Before the stab, the distance between you and the assailant is relatively long and sufficient for a kick.

As the aggressor advances to attack, deliver a kick to the center of his body, while moving your upper body back and thrusting your hip forward. The exact point of impact depends on the timing of the kick and the angle of the assailant's body during the stab. Here, the photograph shows a kick to the solar plexus.

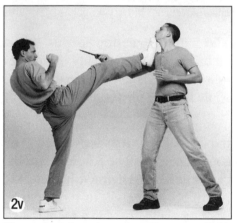

If your kick is executed earlier, you will hit the attacker's chin. An "explosive" switch of heels in place will create a faster kick.

In this technique, it is essential to tilt your upper body sharply back but without shifting your center of gravity backwards, while at the same time delivering a powerful, high, long-range kick. The kick is a combination of a regular (front) kick and swinging the straight leg upward.

Because of the way the kick is executed, it can be aimed at any place in the center of the assailant's body, starting from his groin and up to chin level. If you are wearing hard, pointed shoes, you can kick with your toes; otherwise, kick with the ball of your foot or with your heel.

*Variation: Conditions permitting, you can execute this technique with a body turn, switching the position of your heels in place, with an explosive movement. (See previous technique: **Stab, Oriental Hold – Kick to the Chin**.)*

Note: For our purposes, the "center of the body" means a vertical line passing through the center of body from the head down. Its location varies according to the angle of the opponent's body. The attacker's body should be viewed as a silhouette. Generally, wherever the center line is on the silhouette is considered to be the "center of the body" for defensive purposes. Of course, this line shifts as the relative position between the attacker and the defender changes.

Stab, Straight Hold – Regular Kick to Armpit

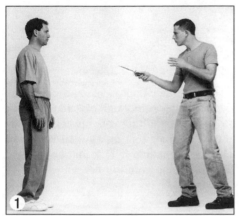

Before the stab, the distance between you and the assailant is relatively long and sufficient for a kick.

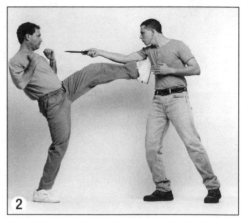

As the assailant advances with his attack, execute a regular kick with your left leg to the armpit of the hand holding the knife, tilting your upper body sharply back.

In this technique, as in the previous one, tilt your upper body sharply back, simultaneously thrusting your pelvis forward and kicking the assailant in the armpit. The defense is executed from the neutral (passive) starting stance and the kicking (left) leg is aligned with the stabbing (right) hand. The armpit is a sensitive, stationary area and is therefore relatively easy to attack. Depending on distance and timing, a highly skilled combatant can land a kick elsewhere on the stabbing arm, e.g., on the wrist, forearm, or elbow.

Note: These last two techniques, essentially, are identical. Apart from your personal preference as to which leg delivers the kick, the choice between them depends on the angle from which the assailant attacks, relative to your position: if the attacker is diagonally to your right, you will kick him in the armpit with your right foot. If he is diagonally to your left, kick with your left leg, aiming at the center of his body. This demonstrates a basic principle of Krav Maga: **Choose the defense or the attack according to the relative positions of your body and the assailant's**.

Stab, Straight Hold – Lateral Body Defense and Kick

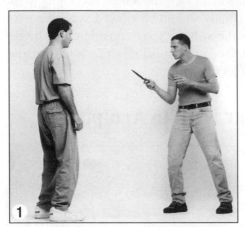

Before the stab there is a safe distance between you and the assailant, meaning that he must advance in order to stab you.

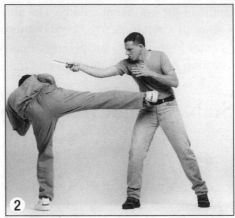

As the assailant approaches and stabs, leap diagonally sideways and forward in a quick stomping step, tilting your upper body sideways and turning your chest toward the ground. Deliver a roundhouse kick to the attacker's solar plexus or groin.

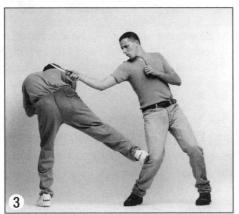

The roundhouse kick is followed by a side kick to the assailant's knee, or by immediately distancing yourself from the assailant.

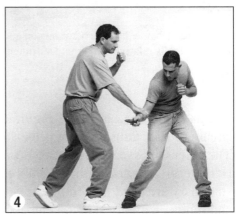

If you decide to control and further counterattack, act according to the new situation created. For example, grab the assailant's attacking arm with your (right) hand, while preparing a punch.

This technique is most suitable against an assailant who charges forward with great momentum, as it takes you away from the line of attack. It is also convenient to implement when you are moving, i.e., while shifting your weight from foot to foot, or when you lose your balance. It is especially convenient when your kicking leg is in front.

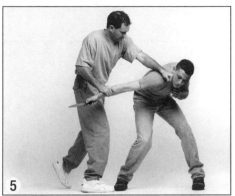

5

Punch the assailant's chin with your left (rear) fist. If he is wearing a coat or a long-sleeved shirt, it is most convenient to grab his sleeve.

Your head leads your body movements: in this case, tilting your upper body such that your chest is parallel to the ground (not a lateral tilt) and advancing with a quick skipping step diagonally forward. The direction and distance of that movement should correspond to the depth of the attacker's advance and will depend on the length of the attacker's body and limbs compared to yours. It may also depend on the timing involved between the attack and your defense responding to it. For example, if you have long legs or your timing is late, you can move sideways or even diagonally backwards. If your legs are comparatively short or your timing is early, you should advance further forward.

At the start of your body movement, bring your right hand near your neck, for greater safety, in order to deflect or stop a possible attack to that area. You should aim the roundhouse kick at the assailant's solar plexus, stomach, or groin, according to his position during the stab.

Any further action will depend on the effectiveness of your initial counterattacks. If necessary, you can either kick the assailant again or grab the hand that is holding the knife and counterattack with your other hand. **Remember**: The action is over **only when you have completely neutralized the danger in all its aspects**!

Variations: Execute one kick only (roundhouse or side kick) and follow up by taking control of the attacking hand, and then counterattack. Another option: Move away quickly after your first or second counterattack.

A Real-Life Story

A security man trained in Krav Maga was attacked by a powerfully built terrorist. The terrorist charged him suddenly and repeatedly attempted to stab him in the neck with a 16" (40 cm) long knife. The security man executed a simple defense against these attacks, blocking the assailant's forearm with his own as it moved in towards him. He then shoved the terrorist backwards, cocked his weapon, and shot him.

Stab, Straight Hold – Side Kick

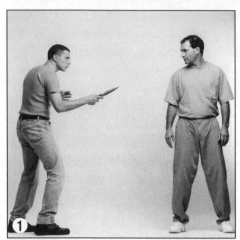

The assailant comes from your side. At this distance, he has to advance before stabbing.

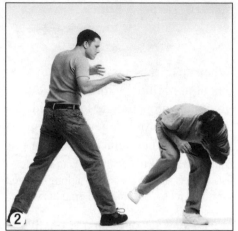

The assailant advances in order to stab. Lean sideways, lower your torso, and simultaneously advance as necessary. In this example, you advance by switching your front foot with your rear foot. Your hand (the one nearer the attacker) is ready to defend if needed.

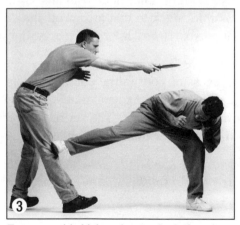

Execute a side kick to the attacker's front knee or to his lower ribs, in order to stop him while he is still at a distance and keep the knife away from you. Your base leg and upper body are bent. By lowering yourself under and away from the attack, you achieve your body defense.

This technique combines a body defense and a stopping attack with the correct timing. The upper torso leans sideways, the hip of the kicking leg shoots towards the assailant as you kick him. This will create a strong kick, and at the same time constitute a body defense for vital areas of your body (e.g., upper torso). The side kick is the action which stops the advancing attacker while he is still at a distance. It is performed while advancing, closing the initial distance in accordance with the timing of the entire action.

The different possibilities for moving, in order to place yourself at the best distance for your attack are the following: back-crossing the legs, switching heels, kicking from where you stand, or even executing side kicks while retreating. Two **vulnerable points** to hit on the attacker's body are the forward knee, and the lower rib area and solar plexus.

In the interest of **safety**, you can use your forward hand to deflect the stabbing hand. However, it is doubtful whether this move is really necessary. In case of a **sudden, surprise attack** you might perform such a defensive measure, if only as a reflex action. At the same time that you bend your upper body, deliver the side kick explosively.

When an assailant comes from the front, you can apply this technique starting from a neutral position, with a slight advance or retreat and a body turn, which will bring you to the proper angle for the side kick. After the above action, proceed with other kicks or, in order to neutralize any danger, grab and gain control of the attacker's hand and counterattack with your rear (left) hand, or simply put yourself at a safe distance from the assailant.

Note: The last two techniqes can also be applied against the other modes of knife attacks that are described in this chapter.

Defenses against Slashing Attack

Anyone who uses this form of attack establishes a more complicated fighting scenario from the outset. Usually, the assailant's objective is first to cut and harm (even superficially), and then to plunge the knife into vital parts of your body.

Many of the principles that were previously detailed, especially against attacks in a straight hold, also apply to the various defenses against slashing knife attacks:

- **Throwing a small object**: At an early stage, **when the assailant intends to attack,** you can throw a small object such as a bunch of keys, a watch, or a wallet at his face or eyes, in order to distract and startle him. This technique is demonstrated in Chap. 7: **Using Everyday Objects as Defensive Weapons**. Follow with the proper advance, and kick the assailant in the groin.

- **Defense by leaning sideways and executing a roundhouse kick**: As demonstrated against a straight stab and performed in the correct direction and at the proper time.

- **Kicking defense, tilting your upper body back**: For example, regular kick to the center line of the assailant's body or to his head, as demonstrated in photographs a&b (see next page); or a side kick as shown in the techniques against straight stab.

- **Forearm defense to stop the attacking hand**: Tilt your upper body back to avoid the first slash. (See photograph c.) Once the knife has passed from one side to the other, and as it comes back, defend with one or both of your forearms against the attacking arm, blocking the attack. If need be, **you can also stop the first slash** with a forearm block, as shown in photograph d. (These principles are also demonstrated in defending against slash attack in Chap. 8: **Short Stick against Knife Attack**.)

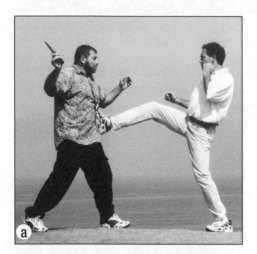

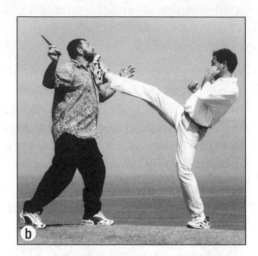

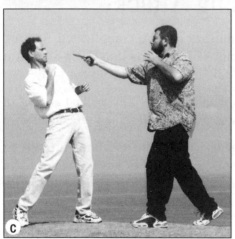

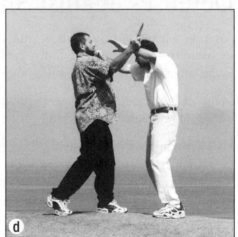

Note: The slashing attack is more sophisticated and harder to defend against with hand defenses, especially against a skilled assailant whose slashing movements are short and fast. As you block the attack, or as soon as possible thereafter, **you must counterattack to neutralize the assailant**.

Knife Attack: Special Situations

Assailant Attacking from Behind

Anyone who comes at you and attacks with a knife **will most likely stab you**, and should be considered as someone who is **intending to kill**! Pertaining to an assailant who attacks from behind and due to the inherent "element of surprise" that exists in this situation, it must be clearly understood that he may be extremely difficult to handle.

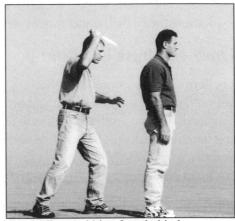

An assailant stabbing from behind.

Against a determined assailant, you basically have the following choices: (1) Escape. (2) Defend, counterattack to thwart the attack, and retreat at the first moment that it is safe to do so. (3) Neutralize the assailant with effective defenses and aggressive counterattacks.

Due to the severity of the danger, do not refrain from taking any action or executing any attack that could save your life or hurt the assailant, including those attacks that ordinary people may consider "out of line" or extremely ferocious. It is permitted (as well as recommended) to make use of **any nearby object** that might help you achieve this goal. (See Chap. 7: **Using Everyday Objects as Defensive Weapons**.)

Advance feeling

If you sense, in any way: by sight, hearing or "gut feeling" that you are about to be attacked from behind, you can act in one of the following ways.

- **Attacking to the rear**: While glancing back and bending your upper body forward, which can be accompanied by a step forward, as needed, execute a kick straight to the rear. In Krav Maga this kick is called: "**Defensive kick backwards**." It is performed straight backwards, in much the same way as a horse or bull kicks with his rear leg.

- **Turning to the rear while executing a defensive action**: While turning around, move slightly away and execute a forearm defense. This will usually place the attacker alongside you. In this position, you must defend and counterattack according to the angle and type of stab. As early as possible, counterattack decisively with an appropriate technique.

- **Moving away**: Having sensed the approaching attack, you should distance yourself from the assailant. Depending on the circumstances, your direction of movement shall be forward, diagonally forward, or sideways. While moving, look backwards, and then, as quickly as possible, turn to the aggressor and "welcome" him with a kick or a hand defense and then counterattack, as demonstrated by the techniques described in this chapter.

Once you have been stabbed...

The knife has penetrated your body. Usually, during the first few moments you will not realize that you have been stabbed, but rather will feel an ordinary impact and pain as if you had just been punched. Removing the knife may cause greater bleeding and damage, including internal hemorrhage, and should be done **only by a qualified person**. Moreover, if the knife is removed, the assailant can use it again! Note that our main objective here will be **to prevent the aggressor from stabbing you again**.

Once you realize that you have been attacked from behind, as though somebody struck you, you should assume that the assailant is using a weapon such as a knife, ax, or similar object. React quickly: move fast, taking three or four steps away from the assailant while turning towards him. If you do not move away fast enough, you will probably be attacked again and again, and **the harm will be much greater**. Your direction of movement should be forward or sideways, according to circumstances. While moving away, look back to see the assailant and take action against him, according to the distance and his actions, using the techniques described in this chapter. Always maintain your fighting spirit: do not panic, and do not quit!

If you feel that you cannot stand up, you can still move away in another direction by falling to the ground. Fall close to the attacker, land on your side, and from this position attack the assailant with kicks from the ground, preferably with the heels, to his knees or groin.

Even after being stabbed once, a well-trained expert can turn quickly towards the assailant and execute defenses and attacks, as circumstances dictate. **The important thing is to remain focused on surviving the incident**. Many victims of knife attacks have survived despite the numerous wounds that were inflicted during the violent encounter. To their credit, these individuals kept on fighting and **did not quit**. Therefore, do not lose your will to fight, conquer, and survive, even if you have received one or more stab wounds.

You Are Carrying a Gun, and the Assailant Attacks you with a Sharp or Blunt Object

If a crazed attacker assaults you when your gun is holstered or not otherwise available for immediate use, your empty-hand defense training must be employed to save your body from immediate critical injury. Most attackers can close a gap of fifteen to twenty feet before a defender is ready to utilize higher force options such as a handgun or baton! Many law-enforcement officers around the world have unfortunately lost their lives as tragic proof of this fact...

In experiments with a knife-wielding assailant who was standing less than twenty feet (six meters) from, and bursting towards an officer who was aware of the danger facing him, it was proven that any attempts that the officer makes to retrieve and operate his (or her) firearm will be made in vain, and that he (or she) will ultimately be stabbed several times! This is due to the time needed in order to react effectively, which is composed of the time needed to process the information about the attack and make a decision to draw the gun from its holster, plus the time needed to aim and fire. This time may vary between 1.5 and 3 seconds, during which the assailant can practically operate undisturbed. Therefore, even if you carry a gun, you must practice hand and foot defenses and counterattacks in order to survive an attack at close range, as detailed above.

Having neutralized the initial danger by performing leg techniques (kicks) or using your hands and executing initial counterattacks, and, if possible, having established a safe distance by moving away, only then you may be able to safely and effectively draw your gun. (See photograph a.) If you are an officer or soldier carrying a submachine gun or assault rifle, and are attacked at close range, you should be able to use the weapon to defend yourself and counterattack. In effect, you are first using the gun as an impact weapon (blunt object) to redirect or block the initial attack and counterattack: striking with the gun (as in photograph c) or delivering a kick, and only then rendering the gun operable as a firearm, if needed, to neutralize the assailant.

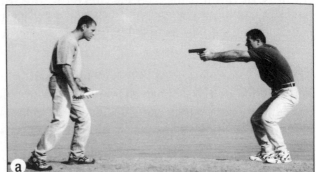

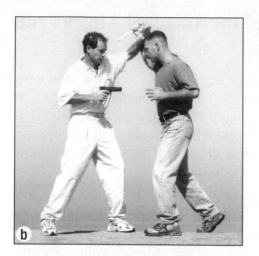
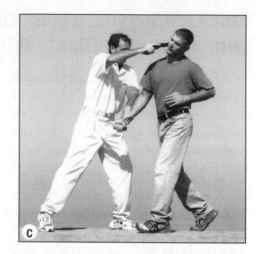

There have been cases in which a stabber in a state of delirium (possibly under the influence of drugs, sudden insanity, religious fanaticism, etc.) continued to attack even after he had been shot several times, as he did not feel pain and was unaware that he had been shot (especially if he was shot with a small-caliber round). This illustrates the tremendous determination of a knife-wielding aggressor. Therefore, you must be prepared to defend and counterattack with your hands and legs if you do not have the opportunity to utilize higher force options. (See photograph b.) In fact, your gun may only serve as an accessory; **do not rely solely on your gun** as an all-powerful "magic" tool to save the day. You must be a total warrior, with or without weapons such as mace, O.C. spray, batons, and firearms.

Summary

When executing a knife attack, the assailant definitely intends to kill or inflict great bodily injury. He exerts power and speed in the attack, and is liable to stab several times. In hand defense techniques, the basic principle is to deflect or stop the attack, preventing reuse of the weapon, and, as early as possible, to counterattack in order to neutralize the aggressor. When necessary, the opponent should be disarmed.

Kicking techniques against knife attacks are effective at long range. Their purpose is to hurt and stop the assailant before he achieves a closer range that may endanger your safety.

The techniques described in this chapter shall be applied only when you have no other choice. If you do have a choice, it is preferable that you simply flee the scene or, if this is impossible, use a dedicated weapon (such as a gun) or an improvised one (iron bar, stick, chair, etc.) to aid in your defense.

Defense against Impending Threat with a Knife

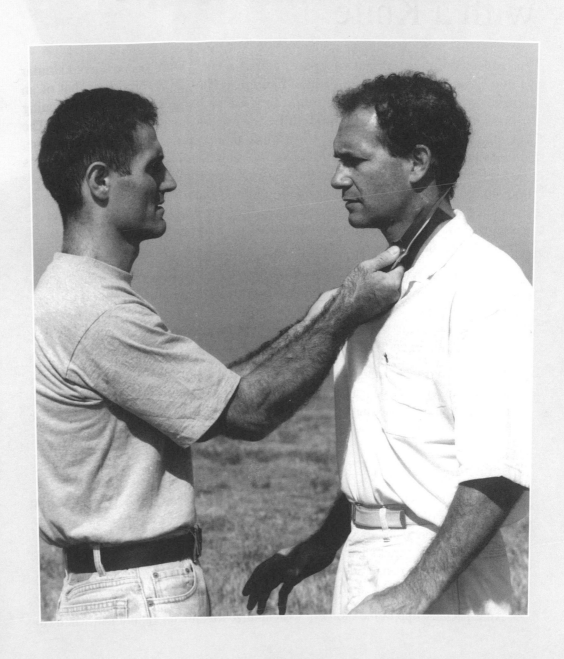

Chapter 2

Defense against Impending Threat with a Knife

The objective of an assailant who poses a threat with a knife is considered si... to that of someone threatening with a handgun. His aim differs from that... attacker who is actually stabbing or slashing with a knife. The person thre... with a knife **wishes to achieve something** by way of threat and intimidat... assailant's goal may be to obtain information, money, property, or someth... or even just to move the victim from one location to another. He usually prese... the knife in an aggressive and threatening manner, or holds it against the victim's body in order to instill fear and to gain the victim's immediate cooperation, with no resistance whatsoever. Therefore, the essence of the problem is the threat and the positioning of the knife, which generally does not make any significant movements relative to the victim's body.

The assailant may threaten his victim from different ranges (close, medium, and long) and from various directions and angles. He can present his weapon at different heights, and may hold it against the victim at different parts of the body in order to gain control over him. The assailant is also liable to grab the victim by his clothing, his arm, his hair, or another part of the body, all in order to impose his will.

Historically, our techniques for handling an impending threat with a knife were developed, based in large part on the fundamental principles for neutralizing threat from a handgun, defenses against an attack with a knife, and defenses against a stab with a bayoneted rifle.

Operation Principles

- Perform the technique **as quickly and as soon as possible** after the initial perception of the threat. Remember that a moving knife (a stab or a slash) presents a more dangerous scenario, while a motionless knife typifies a different, less dangerous threat. The more time that passes from the moment the threat begins, the more dangerous the situation is liable to become, and the more likely it is to deteriorate into an actual knife attack (stabbing or slashing).

- An especially opportune moment to neutralize the threat is a moment **when the**

46

Defense against Impending Threat with a Knife

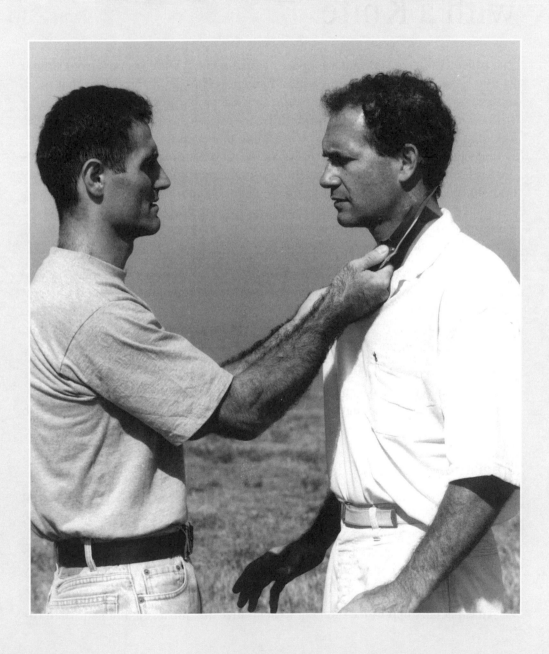

Defense against Impending Threat with a Knife

The objective of an assailant who poses a threat with a knife is considered similar to that of someone threatening with a handgun. His aim differs from that of an attacker who is actually stabbing or slashing with a knife. The person threatening with a knife **wishes to achieve something** by way of threat and intimidation. The assailant's goal may be to obtain information, money, property, or something else, or even just to move the victim from one location to another. He usually presents the knife in an aggressive and threatening manner, or holds it against the victim's body in order to instill fear and to gain the victim's immediate cooperation, with no resistance whatsoever. Therefore, the essence of the problem is the threat and the positioning of the knife, which generally does not make any significant movements relative to the victim's body.

The assailant may threaten his victim from different ranges (close, medium, and long) and from various directions and angles. He can present his weapon at different heights, and may hold it against the victim at different parts of the body in order to gain control over him. The assailant is also liable to grab the victim by his clothing, his arm, his hair, or another part of the body, all in order to impose his will.

Historically, our techniques for handling an impending threat with a knife were developed, based in large part on the fundamental principles for neutralizing threat from a handgun, defenses against an attack with a knife, and defenses against a stab with a bayoneted rifle.

Operation Principles

- Perform the technique **as quickly and as soon as possible** after the initial perception of the threat. Remember that a moving knife (a stab or a slash) presents a more dangerous scenario, while a motionless knife typifies a different, less dangerous threat. The more time that passes from the moment the threat begins, the more dangerous the situation is liable to become, and the more likely it is to deteriorate into an actual knife attack (stabbing or slashing).

- An especially opportune moment to neutralize the threat is a moment **when the**

46

assailant's attention is slightly distracted. For example, when he is talking and giving orders, or listening to the victim's pleas for mercy.

- In response to a defensive movement, the assailant is liable **to react reflexively** by retracting the hand holding the knife in order to use it to stab or slash at the victim. He is also liable to stab or slash immediately, or to shove or otherwise attack the victim with a kick or with his free hand. The basic techniques against threat with a knife take into consideration such "natural" and predictable reactions of the assailant to your defensive action.

- Most of the defensive techniques for neutralizing a threat with a knife from close range, and especially when the assailant is grabbing the victim, are based on the underlying principles and defensive techniques against a handgun threat: (1) **Active defense with the hand** coupled with a corresponding **body defense**. (2) **Gaining control of the weapon or, actually the hand that is holding it**, while advancing towards the attacker. (3) **Delivering a forceful counterattack**. (4) Concluding by **disarming the assailant or moving away to a safe distance**.

- Generally, at your first possible opportunity, you need to distance yourself as far as possible from the scene of the encounter. It should be noted that the specific techniques for neutralizing a threat with a knife are often performed **without disarming the assailant** (i.e., without taking the knife). This approach is generally recommended, as in many cases it is more efficient and effective to secure the attacker's hand holding the knife, deliver forceful counterattacks, and retreat from the danger zone, than to try to take the knife from the assailant.

- The defensive actions comprising the techniques for neutralizing a threat with a knife from a relatively **long range** are based on the underlying principles and defensive techniques against straight stabbing-type attacks with a stick or bayoneted rifle. These principles are: First **deflecting** the threat with an open-handed slap and, when necessary, leaning forward and turning the body, and then **kicking** the adversary.

The following are examples of how to deal correctly with various threats posed by a knife. You should first practice the basic techniques, and then, based on what you have learned, practice dealing with different threat scenarios that are variations of, but closely resemble, the basic techniques. Remember that in a real-life situation, the assailant's actions are not exactly predictable. Therefore, after learning the basic exercises, practice in realistic, pressure-filled training sessions in order to experience and become acquainted with a wide range of potential dangers, which are not specifically addressed in this chapter. This approach to training should be applied to **all subjects** dealt with in this book.

Long-distance Threat from the Front

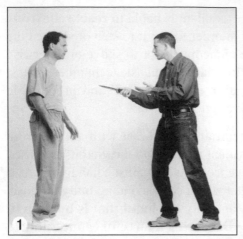

1

You have become aware of a knife threat from the front. The assailant is relatively far away, and is holding the knife in front of him.

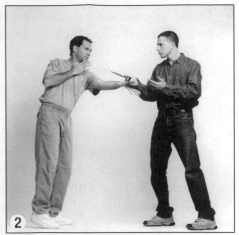

2

In the most economical way possible, deflect the danger to the side with an open-handed strike (with fingers outstretched) to the back of the assailant's hand. This defensive hand movement leads the body in a slight turn that serves as a body defense, and a slight lean forward is to be executed when needed in order to increase the range covered by your hand defense (deflection).

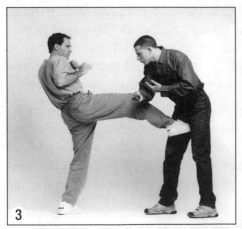

3

Continue with a regular kick to the groin, while moving your torso backwards and away from the knife. Conclude by fleeing the scene or by continuing to neutralize the attacker as described in the following stages. It is possible that the sudden strike to deflect the knife, or the strong kick, will cause the assailant to drop the knife.

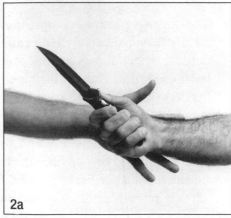

2a

Close-up, photograph 2: Strike to the back of the assailant's hand.

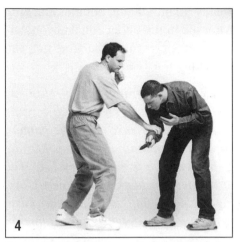

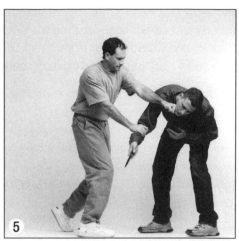

If you choose not to leave, it is suggested that you do the following: As you retract your leg from delivering the kick, grab the assailant's hand that is holding the knife (near his elbow) with your near (right) hand, and shift your weight onto it.

Continue with a punch and additional counter-attacks as necessary, e.g., knees or kicks.

Deflecting the assailant's hand resembles the deflection performed in the defense technique against a stab with a stick or bayoneted rifle. The defender's hand is positioned with the thumb pointing up and the pinkie down, while the palm of the hand is open with fingers outstretched. The defender's hand moves diagonally forward to hit the target, which is the assailant's hand holding the knife.

The defensive hand movement is as economical as possible, proceeding in a straight line to the side of the assailant's hand and slapping it horizontally to the side. When the knife is held much higher and is in closer proximity to your face, you will have to strike with your hand in a different (vertical) position. In this case, all your fingers shall be held close together, pointing upward.

Between the deflection and the kick you will usually step explosively, in place or while advancing slightly forward, as necessary, so that your weight will be quickly transferred to your base foot. This will also serve to shorten the distance to the target, if necessary, as well as help to facilitate the fastest and strongest kick possible from your original "neutral" stance. It is usually recommended to kick with the foot opposite the deflecting hand. Hit the assailant's groin using a regular front-kick with the instep or, preferably, with the ball of your foot.

In order to prepare yourself for realistic confrontations, you should also practice the tactic of **rapidly leaving the scene of danger immediately after kicking the assailant**. In reality, if this is not possible, then continue as demonstrated here with the next stages of grabbing and controlling the assailant's hand, counterattacking again, and finish by disarming the assailant. After the initial deflection and counter-attack, considerable attention must be given to objects present in the area, that can be used to further assist you in defending or attacking the assailant.

Variations: If the assailant is beside or behind you, threatening from a relatively long distance, the technique is essentially identical. Such a technique will include striking and deflecting the assailant's hand in an outside defense using the palm of your hand or the inner (bony) part of your forearm, continuing by leaning in the opposite direction from the knife, and kicking the assailant as fast as possible. The appropriate kick will usually be a **side kick** *or a* **defensive back-kick**. *If necessary, you can kick the assailant without performing the deflecting action. In this case, great emphasis is placed on performing a significant* **body defense** *in conjunction with the appropriate kick.*

Threat from the Front, when the Knife is Out of Reach

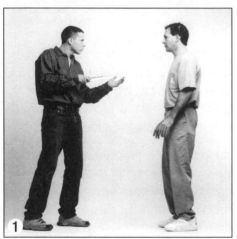

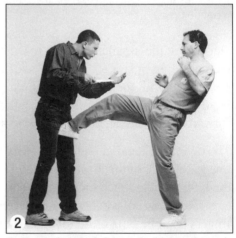

You are faced with a knife threat from an assailant standing at medium or long distance. This situation resembles the previous one, except that although the assailant is close enough, the knife is held at a distance that makes it difficult for you to reach the hand that is holding it.

Deliver a fast, forceful regular kick to the groin while leaning backwards with your torso. If possible, leave the scene quickly. If not, continue attacking the assailant in order to incapacitate him, rendering him unable to use the knife.

This technique resembles the previous one, except for the deflection movement. A highly opportune moment to perform this technique is while you are feigning cooperation and pretending to obey the assailant's orders. (For example, when you are pretending to take your wallet out of your pocket.)

Threat from the Front, at Short Range

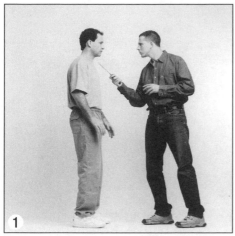

You are faced with a threat from a knife held very close to your throat or elsewhere on your upper body.

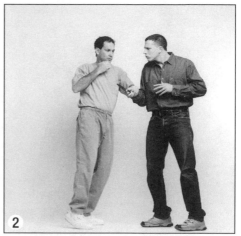

Begin with a defensive hand movement and proceed with a body turn. Redirect the knife horizontally, by moving and grabbing the assailant in the vicinity of the wrist of his hand that is holding the knife. When you touch the assailant's wrist, your thumb should be pointing down and your index finger up. Your weight is transferred diagonally forward, to the side of the deflecting hand.

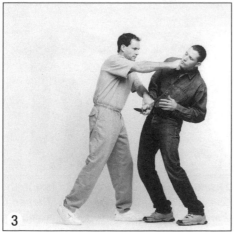

Advance on the same foot as the deflecting hand, transferring your weight so as to apply pressure to the assailant's hand, downwards and to the side. Attack forcefully with a straight punch and put pressure on the knife hand, straightening your elbow. It is then possible to attack the assailant again, or shove him backwards as you move quickly away from him, and leave the scene.

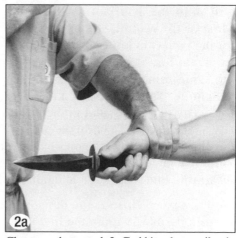

Close-up, photograph 2: Grabbing the assailant's wrist while deflecting it sideways.

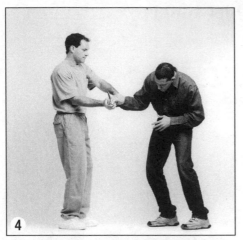

If you choose not to move away, possible further action may be to grab the assailant's hand with both your hands as shown, and make a slight movement backwards, putting yourself in a better position to deliver a strong kick.

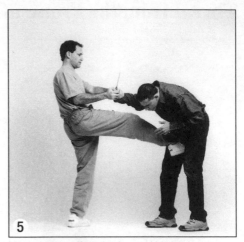

Kick the assailant in the groin.

This technique is based on that used for *Threat from the Front, from a Distance* (see Chap. 4: **Neutralizing a Threat at Gunpoint**), but here you will grab the assailant by the wrist. Most of the neutralization techniques for the variety of knife threats from the front, at close range, will be based on the same principles of this particular technique. They consist of a hand defense (by deflecting and grabbing the adversary's wrist), a body defense (by turning and moving diagonally forward), gaining control of the hand holding the knife (by grasping it and pressing it diagonally downward), attacking the assailant, disarming him (optional), and quickly leaving the scene of danger.

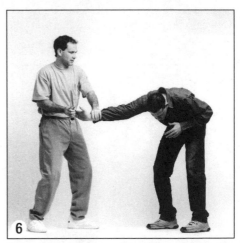

Disarm your adversary as described in the technique: *Stab, Oriental Hold – Diagonal Forearm Defense*. (See previous chapter.)

Note: In some close-range threat situations, if the assailant is not grabbing you, it is still possible to apply the first technique: deflect the threat, kick your adversary, and quickly leave the scene.

Threat to the Throat, from the Front

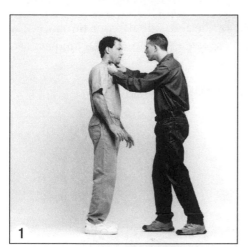

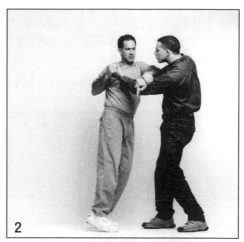

The assailant has put a knife to the right side of your throat. You were unable to prevent this situation as it developed. He has also grabbed your clothes, in order to gain better control over you.

Similar to the previous technique, the appropriate hand (in this case, your left) redirects the knife away from your throat by deflecting and grabbing the assailant's wrist, moving as economically and as fast as possible. At the same time, execute a body defense (turn) and transfer your weight diagonally forward, thereby creating a safety distance between your throat and the knife.

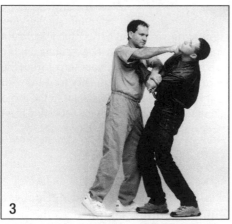

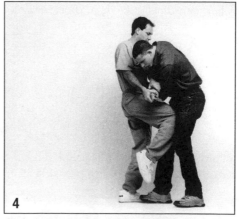

Advance on the same foot as the hand (left), grabbing the assailant's wrist, and attack him with a straight punch while pressing diagonally down on the hand holding the knife.

As shown in the previous technique, deflect the assailant's hand, and grab it. Proceed with a body turn, and advance diagonally forward.

Grab the hand holding the knife with your other hand too, in order to gain better control over the assailant's hand, and attack again with a knee kick to the groin. Continue as previously described for disarming, or shove the assailant backwards and leave the scene quickly.

Counterattack quickly and forcefully. The pressure on the hand holding the knife should be directed diagonally sideways and down, and towards the assailant's body.

The knife could be placed at either the right or the left side of your throat. For a situation where the knife is placed at the left side, see the following technique.

Threat to the Throat, Knife Facing Inward

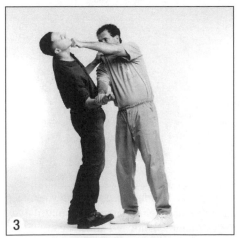

The assailant is holding you for better control (from his point of view) and putting the knife to your throat. This resembles the previous technique, except that the knife is facing inwards.

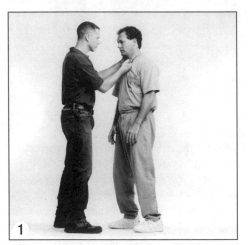

Continue to approach the assailant, and strike him. Conclude with additional counterattacks, shove the opponent, and either distance yourself from him or disarm him.

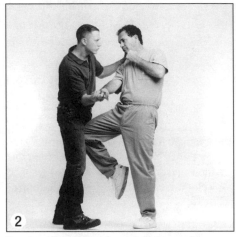

Implement the basic technique, using your **right hand**. Grab and deflect the assailant's wrist while simultaneously executing a body turn in order to distance your throat from the knife. As you move diagonally forward with your right leg, kick the assailant in the groin and straighten the elbow of the deflecting hand (your right hand).

It is clear that an inward deflection with the left hand, similar to the previous technique, would cause your throat to be cut. Therefore, the basic defensive technique will be executed with the **right hand**. Deflect the knife as you grab the assailant's wrist with your right hand. Protect your body by distancing it from the knife, shifting your weight diagonally forward, and delivering an attack with your knee.

If needed, it is possible to first counterattack with a straight punch as you advance diagonally forward on your right leg, and then to deliver a knee strike to the assailant's groin with your rear (left) leg.

Variations:

- *Deflect and grab the attacker's wrist with your right hand, distancing yourself from the knife, and quickly grab with the left hand as well, securing your hold by cupping the assailant's hand that is holding the knife. This is much safer and, at the same time, you may execute a series of counterattacks with your knee. This resembles the technique used against gun threat,* **Diagonal Threat from the Front, from a Distance – Entry on "Live" Side**. *(Chap. 4:* **Neutralizing a Threat at Gunpoint**.*)*

- *An outside defense performed with your left hand may also be possible in some cases. Counterattack simultaneously with a punch, performing the same body defense (moving diagonally forward with your right leg), and deflect the assailant's wrist (with your left). In this variation the grab (control) is performed relatively later than in the demonstrated technique.*

Threat from Behind, with Shoulder Grab

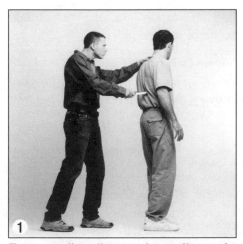

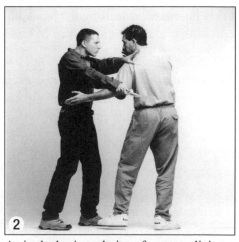

From a medium distance, the assailant grabs you by the clothes, near your shoulder, and puts a knife to your back. His intention may be only to threaten you, or perhaps to take you somewhere else.

As in the basic technique for neutralizing a handgun threat from behind, deflect the hand holding the weapon, and at the same time execute a body turn and advance forcefully towards your opponent. (See defense techniques against handgun, e.g., **Threat from Behind, at Close Range**.)

This technique is almost identical to the one for neutralizing a handgun threat from behind; we suggest that you review this section of the book at this time.

The deflecting hand "pulls" the body into a turn, followed by a forward burst towards the assailant. If the assailant shoves you forward with his hand (the same hand that is grabbing your clothing), or if you feel that the location of the shoving hand or the knife will make it difficult for you to execute the body turn in the direction shown here (left), then perform a reverse technique: turn to the right while deflecting and grabbing the assailant's forearm with your right hand.

Having deflected the assailant's hand, your hand moves diagonally forward. Then, in a sweeping movement, catch his forearm (of the hand holding the knife) near the elbow. At the same time, execute an elbow strike to the assailant's jaw or throat area. Note that your elbow strike moves horizontally inward and forward, as if penetrating the intended target.

Here too, as in the previous technique, the principles are the same: hand and body defense, controlling the hand that is holding the weapon, attacking the assailant forcefully, and disarming him or leaving the scene of danger.

Variation: If the assailant does not grab you, in most cases you can deflect his hand by striking it with your forearm, simultaneously taking a quick step, leaning forward and delivering a defensive kick backwards, applying the principles used in the first technique presented in this chapter.

A Real-Life Story

Avi, an Israeli instructor of Krav Maga, was strolling along the Copa Cabana Beach in Rio de Janeiro. He was approached by three people who intended to rob him. The one on his left put a knife to his throat, the second began fishing for something in his pocket, and the third was standing a few feet away. Avi deflected the hand holding the knife – as exemplified by the relevant techniques in this chapter. As a result of this action, the knife cut the second attacker's face. At the same time, the first assailant who was holding the knife was driven to the ground by two punches. The second attacker, as a result of his injury, slipped and retreated backwards (clutching his face) and the third ran away. The "victim" of the attempted assault retreated quickly in the opposite direction.

Threat from Behind, at Close Range

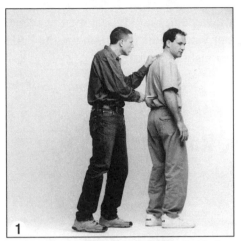

1

The assailant approaches you from behind, at very close range. He grips your shoulder and puts a knife to your back. You cannot turn and take a step to your left **because of the forward pressure being applied to your left shoulder**.

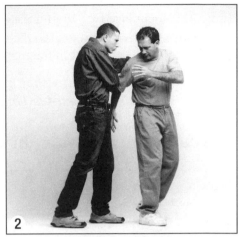

2

As in the previous technique, deflect the assailant's hand and proceed with a quick body turn outward while coming closer to the adversary. The assailant is now very close to you, making it difficult to grab his forearm with your defending arm. Therefore, grab and secure his elbow or upper arm with your other hand, and step onto your right leg towards the assailant.

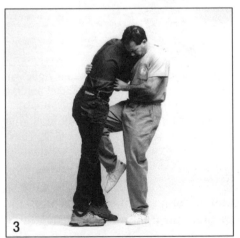

3

Grab the assailant by putting your right arm around him (since you have turned to the right). With your left hand, grab him near the elbow and push the elbow inward. Advance quickly with your left leg, come alongside the assailant, and as you push him backwards, deliver a series of knee strikes to his groin with your right leg.

This technique, quite similar to the previous one, begins by deflecting the hand holding the weapon. The deflection is immediately followed by a body turn and advance on the same foot as the deflecting arm.

Due to the very close range at the outset that brings you beside or behind the assailant, it is very difficult to execute the basic technique of grabbing his forearm with the deflecting arm. The solution is to come very close to the attacker and "embrace" him.

Simultaneously, neutralize the hand holding the knife by grabbing the upper arm near the elbow, clinching the assailant while pushing him backwards.

Finish this technique by shoving the attacker away and quickly leaving the scene, or by using your left hand to grab the forearm or wrist of the hand holding the knife and disarming the assailant in the manner previously demonstrated.

*Variation: In some cases (as shown in the next technique), you could grab the assailant's forearm **with your left hand**, instead of his upper arm.*

Threat from the Side, at Close Range

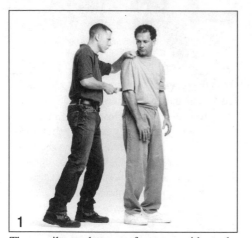

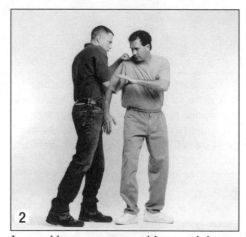

The assailant, who came from your side, grabs you near the shoulder and puts the knife to your ribs, behind your arm. His objective is most likely to rob you. He will be restricting your movement and threatening you with the knife, holding it in such a way that it cannot be easily detected by bystanders.	In a sudden movement, with your right arm held straight down, deflect the hand holding the knife, sending it towards the attacker's stomach while executing a body turn. Your other hand is ready to grab the assailant's forearm as you advance (if necessary) towards him.

As in the basic technique for neutralizing handgun threat from behind or from the side, here too you deflect the threat, execute a body turn in order to create a body defense, and burst towards the assailant. But here, due to the distance and the angle involved, it is difficult to execute an "ordinary" forearm grab with your deflecting arm. Therefore, you must grab the assailant's forearm (of the hand holding the weapon) with your other hand (your left), in order to control his movements and prevent him from withdrawing his hand. Enhance your control by adding your right hand. Attack as soon as possible, making it difficult for your opponent to use his weapon. Finish by disarming the assailant or distancing yourself from him.

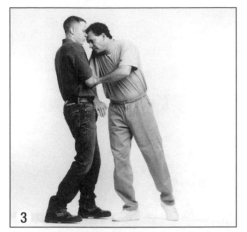

Grab the assailant's forearm, continuing to apply pressure with your deflecting (right) arm. Attack as soon as possible, for example, by delivering a powerful head-butt to a vulnerable spot on the assailant's head or face.

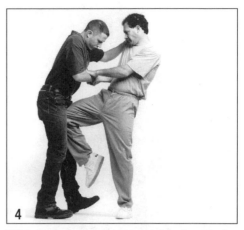

With your deflecting (right) hand, grab the assailant's hand that is holding the knife and knee him in the groin. Continue by distancing yourself from the danger zone or disarming the assailant.

Threat from Behind, Knife at the Throat

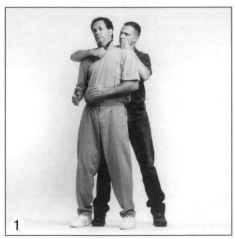

The assailant is behind you, grabs you and puts the knife to your throat.

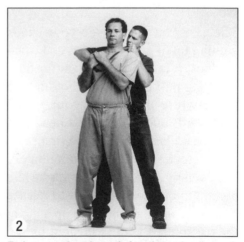

Raise your hands and, forming a hook, grab the area of the assailant's wrist and pull the knife away from your throat while distancing your throat in the opposite direction.

The assailant's objective in this case is to pose a threat to the victim that will deprive him of the ability to resist, whether his ultimate intention might have been robbery or hostage-taking. This defense is based on the fundamental Krav Maga technique of releasing oneself from a head lock (arm-bar choke) from behind.

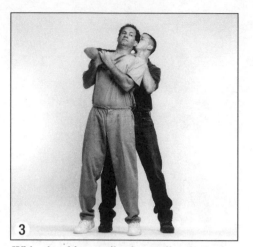

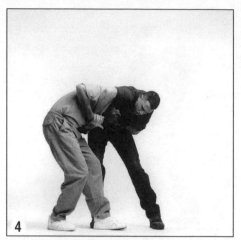

With a head-butt, strike the assailant in the face and distance the knife further by pulling down on his wrist lower. Slightly raise your right shoulder. All this time you are pressing the hand holding the knife strongly to your chest. If necessary, you can strike the assailant's groin during this stage or the previous one.

Continue with a body turn (with your head facing the direction of the opening that has been created) while taking great care that **the knife does not come near your throat**, and get out with your head through the opening.

The assailant cannot see your hands coming up to grab his wrist, and when he does, it is already too late for him. A strong pull on the hand holding the knife while distancing your throat backwards and delivering a head-butt to the assailant's face, is the first stage of the technique. It is immediately followed by a strong turn inward while bending your body in order to release yourself from the hold. The opening in the assailant's hold is created by the

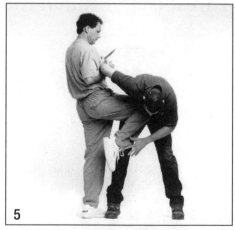

Attack again, with the assailant's hand still held firmly against your chest.

strong pull on his wrist and the swift movement of your body. Your left shoulder should dip to facilitate the escape, and raising your right shoulder helps you to control and limit the assailant's ability to move the knife closer to you.

Note: In general, this is considered a relatively **high-risk technique** and, therefore, should be performed **only as a last resort**! Sometimes it might be worthwhile to wait until your situation changes for the better.

Defending against an Assailant Armed with a Stick

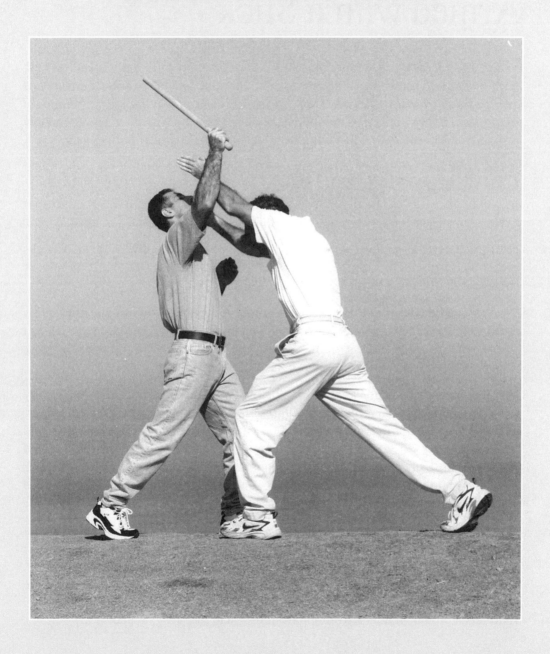

Chapter 3

Defending against an Assailant Armed with a Stick

When using a stick as a weapon, an assailant will usually hold the stick at one end, with one or two hands. Possible attacks with the stick include ***overhead downward swing, forward strike, forward stab, horizontal swing from the side,*** or ***diagonal swing from above***, performed at different heights. There are also other, less commonly utilized attacks such as rising swing from below, either vertical or diagonal.

A highly skilled combatant, depending on the length and weight of the stick, might hold the stick at both ends and use a variety of attack techniques. During the attack, he might also vary his hold on the stick, e.g., pass it from hand to hand or grasp it at one end so that the short, rear part of the stick can also be used for attack.

Note: The defenses against stick attack can also be used effectively against attacks with objects resembling a stick, such as an iron bar, ax, club, baseball bat, hoe, or rifle with or without a bayonet attached.

We must remember that **the fastest and most dangerous part of the stick is its front end**, the end that is being directed at you. The closer we move to the back end of the stick towards the assailant's hands, the less powerful (and therefore less dangerous) the strike will be. This is a basic characteristic of stick attacks.

The defenses against stick attacks include the two types of actions that are usually incorporated into defense techniques: ***hand defenses*** and ***body (evasion) defenses***. The body defenses are based on bursting forward (sometimes in diagonal line) and advancing very close to the assailant. These types of body defenses are directed mainly against strikes in which the assailant swings the stick vertically downward, diagonally downward or horizontally, as one would swing a baseball bat. (See drawings a, e and d.)

With an overhead attack, the hand defenses are based on a **sliding defense** that redirects the stick or the aggressor's forearm (drawings a, b, and e). Against a horizontal attack (drawing d), the principle of the hand defense, after bursting forward, is to **absorb the momentum** from the less dangerous, slower-moving part of the stick or the aggressor's arm. An inside hand defense is a motion that deflects and redirects a whipping attack from the front or a stab (drawings b and c).

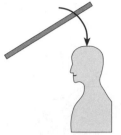
a. Overhead strike from above

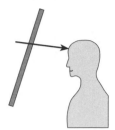
b. Forward strike

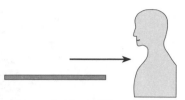
c. Forward stab at different heights

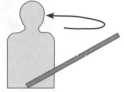
d. Horizontal strike from the side at different heights

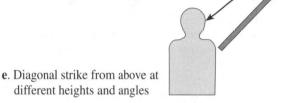
e. Diagonal strike from above at different heights and angles

Overhead Swing – Stabbing Defense to the Inside of the Attack

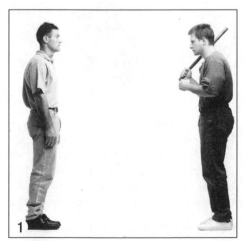

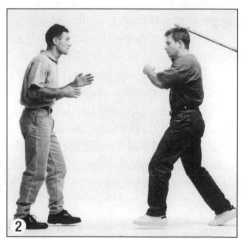

Starting position, i.e., a neutral stance.

Photograph 2: The assailant raises the stick and advances while attacking. Start by raising your hand vertically in a "stabbing defense,"

performed while leaning forward and bursting towards the assailant. The back of the defending hand is facing sideways. Your other hand comes up, ready to attack, while your head is lowered between the shoulders.

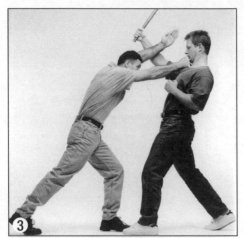

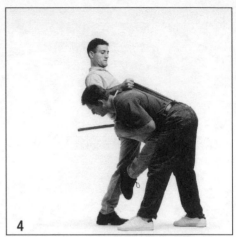

Burst forward with a stabbing defense, sliding your forearm against the inside of the aggressor's forearm. As early as possible, counterattack to the aggressor's throat or chin. Looking at the opponent, your body is tilted diagonally forward, so that an imaginary line can be drawn from your forward hand to your rear heel.

Conclusion of the action, e.g., grabbing the assailant and kneeing him in the groin.

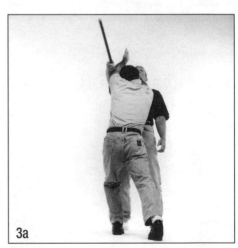

Start with a hand defense (stabbing technique) directed to the inside of the aggressor's forearm. If the attack has taken you by surprise, depending on the timing and manner of the attack, the defense may be made against the stick itself. In either case, the stick or the assailant's arm, once deflected, will slide along the fleshy, outside part of your arm and will be redirected to the outside of your body. The action of the defending hand leads ("pulls") your body into its burst forward.

Situation shown in photograph 3, viewed from behind. The attack slides alongside your arm and body. Your head is held low between your shoulders, your upper arm is touching the back of your ear. You may advance on either foot, depending on the situation, as explained later.

In the stabbing defense, when your arm is rising, the elbow of the defending arm is pointed downward and the arm itself (your biceps) is brought close to your head, which is lowered between your shoulders. This maneuver can also be effective if the assailant is holding the stick **with both hands**, but in this case you must execute the stabbing defense to **the outer side** of the forearm. (See next technique.)

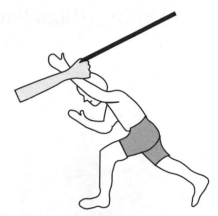

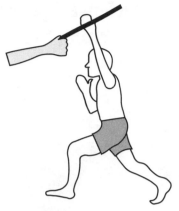

a. Leaning forward: the **correct posture**, which brings your head closer to the assailant and to the less dangerous zone.

b. Standing upright: the **incorrect posture**, in which your head is too far from the assailant.

The body defense is based on bursting forward at the instant the assailant raises his hand to attack. You can use **either foot** in your advance forward. Lunging with the left foot reinforces the hand defense. When bursting forward with your right foot, your body evades the line of attack more effectively.

If you are able to see the attack developing clearly, and it is relatively slow, you will have time to put greater emphasis on the forward burst which, by nature,

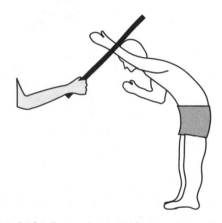

c. Defending against a sudden attack.

will precede the hand defense. Remember that the defense technique and forward burst are to be executed **at the same instant that the adversary raises his hand**, when he is within a range that is liable to endanger you.

Remember: In defending against a sudden attack, advancing your entire body with a forward burst takes too long; emphasis will naturally be on tilting your upper body forward (and also on the hand defense). This reduces the distance to the aggressor and moves the target (i.e., your head) closer to the less dangerous zone of the stick, as illustrated thereafter.

If the attack comes from the front (see drawing b in the introduction to this chapter), it is clear that the defense techniques will be applied against the stick, rather than the assailant's forearm. Keep your head bent low and forward; your defensive hand stab will be directed forward even further than is shown in photographs 2 and 3. (See adjacent drawing.)

Stabbing Defense against Overhead Swing – Standing in Place (Learning Stage)

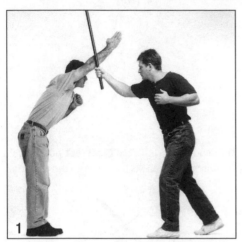

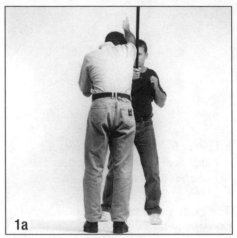

Execute a "stab" to the outer (or inner) side of the attack. Although this is mainly a learning stage illustrating the effectiveness of the defense, this technique is highly useful when you are completely taken by surprise. Your defense is followed by a forward burst and counterattacks.

Situation shown in photograph 1, viewed from behind, emphasizing the sliding path of the attack along the defender's arm and body. The outside, fleshy part of your forearm meets the attack at an acute angle.

In this stage of learning, which illustrates the effectiveness of this technique, we isolate the stabbing defense used against the part of the stick that is closest to the assailant's attacking hand. As a training method, this technique serves to strengthen the hand defenses of the trainee, using attacks of low to medium force with a regular stick, or against a more powerful attack with a padded stick. This is also an example of a fast, reflexive hand defense against a sudden overhead attack with a stick, aimed at your head, when you cannot move forward earlier or fast enough.

The direction and angle of attack dictate whether to use a defense that is directed to the inside or the outside of the attack. Another important factor to be considered is the presence of **additional assailants** and their position relative to yours, e.g., the side from which they are approaching you, etc.

Overhead Swing – Stabbing Defense to the Outside of the Attack

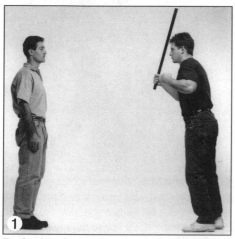

1

Basic situation at the outset: The defender is standing slightly diagonal to the attacker, or in front of him.

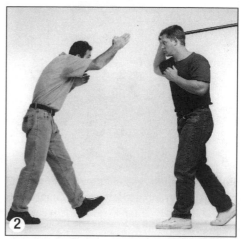

2

The instant the assailant raises his hand and advances to attack, execute a "stabbing defense" (with your right hand), while bursting forward. Your advance is on the foot that is opposite the defending hand.

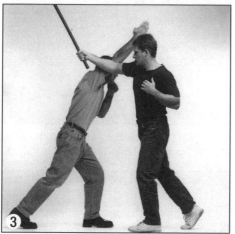

3

Conclusion of the first stage of defense: Execute a "stabbing defense" with your arm, sliding to the outside of the attacker's forearm, while your elbow is facing downward. Your body is tilted diagonally forward, and your head is held low, in between your shoulders. The biceps of the "stabbing" arm is next to your ear (the back of the hand faces out), and the other hand is near your face.

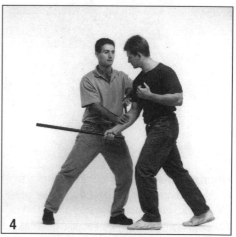

4

Simultaneously with your body turn, follow and meet the attacking hand with both your hands. Your rear leg has moved out of the path of the descending stick.

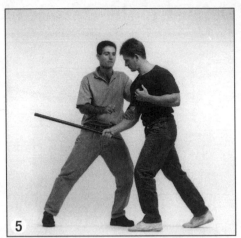

5

Pull the assailant's hand down strongly and change the grabbing (left) hand. Grabbing is especially easy if the assailant is wearing a long-sleeved shirt.

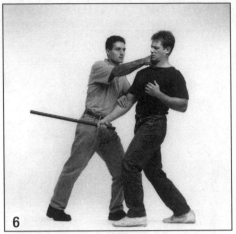

6

Continue attacking with your rear (right) hand, using either a straight punch or a punch that is somewhere between a roundhouse and an uppercut punch, according to the angle between you and the aggressor.

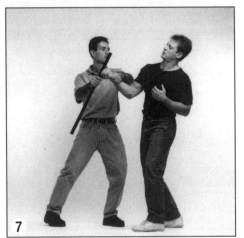

7

Disarm the assailant: hold the attacker's wrist with one hand and the stick with the other. Using a leverage action against the attacker's thumb, rotate the stick downward to break his hold on the stick, and disarm him. If disarming proves difficult, strike the assailant's wrist and the back of his hand with your knee as you rotate the stick downward.

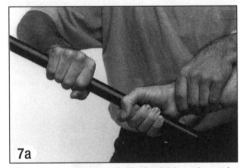

7a

Close-up, photograph 7: Grabbing the wrist and the stick in order to disarm the assailant.

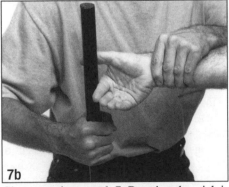

7b

Close-up, photograph 7: Rotating the stick in the assailant's hand will disarm him.

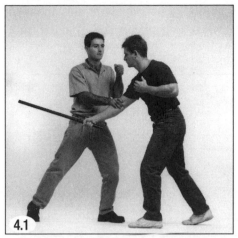

4.1

Rather than in stage 4 where both hands meet and follow the attacking hand, here you will use only one hand (right). Then, while executing a quick body turn, you will send your other (left) hand to attack. As a result of the body turn and hand defense, your rear leg has moved out of the path of the descending stick.

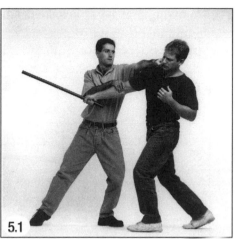

5.1

Grab the attacking arm (or the aggressor's long sleeve) to prevent him from making further use of the stick, and simultaneously counterattack with a straight punch. If the attack swings down with a continuous movement, you will still be able to grab the attacking arm, but only when it is near the assailant's body, and not sooner.

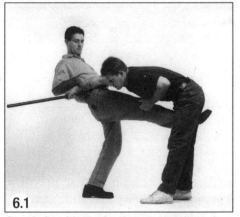

6.1

Conclude with another counterattack, such as a kick to the groin.

When an attacker raises his hand to land a stick on your head, it is usually preferable to burst forward and execute a defense to the **inside** of the attack, as shown above in the first technique in this chapter.

The technique demonstrated here can be applied when you are standing opposite the attacking hand or, alternatively, opposite the aggressor, whenever the situation requires a stabbing defense that will slide along the **outside** of the attacking forearm in order to deflect it. In the latter case, it is necessary to burst diagonally forward. Here, the advance is executed on the foot opposite the defending hand, for a better and quicker body defense, since the direction of the stick attack, especially when it is held in one hand, is diagonally downward.

The following drawings illustrate the different possibilities for applying this approach (defending to the outside of the attacker's arm) when you are attacked from the front, just slightly off-center, or from the side.

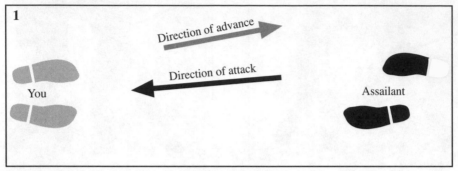

Drawing 1: Standing opposite the aggressor, advance diagonally outward so as to execute the stabbing defense to the outside of the attack. In this situation, when the stick is held in one hand (unless otherwise required), it is usually preferable to apply the first technique: *Overhead Swing – Stabbing Defense to the Inside of the Attack*.

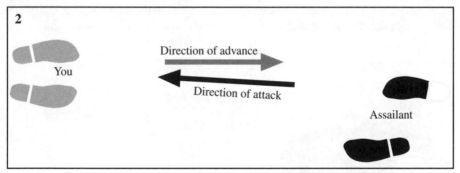

Drawing 2: Application of the current defense is most natural in this position, when standing opposite the attacking hand. The advance shall be straight ahead, as shown in photograph 3.

In defense to the outside of the attack, as shown here, situations may arise in which the same hand and foot should be in front. This may be necessary, for example, against an aggressor attacking from the side, or when you have to move in close behind the assailant for tactical reasons. In this situation, **the attacker's body may actually serve as a shield** against an additional threat, such as a second assailant coming from behind the defender. (For further details, see the technique *Overhead Swing – Stabbing Defense to the outside of the Attack, Advancing with Two Steps*.)

Overhead Swing with Two Hands – Stabbing Defense

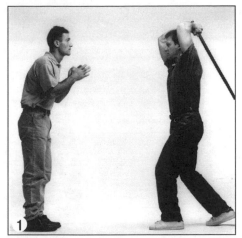

The assailant commences action. Start with a hand defense by "stabbing" and bursting forward.

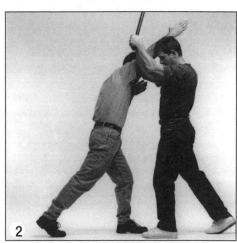

The defense, similar to the previous technique, is carried out against the assailant's forearm or his stick.

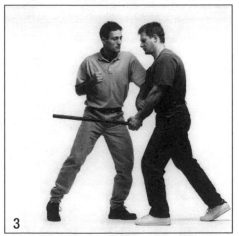

Executing a body turn while moving your rear leg backwards and away from the direction of the descending stick, grab the assailant's hand and apply downward pressure to it.

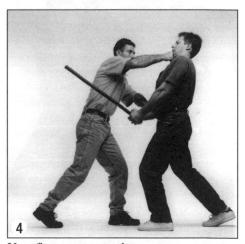

Your first counterattack.

The forward burst and the defense technique are executed similarly to the previous technique. While the assailant's hands continue to move downward, you must execute a body turn, grab his arm, and pin it down with your other hand. You should start your initial counterattack as early as possible.

Variation*: Instead of executing the body turn described in stage 3, you can simply continue by kneeing the assailant's groin with your rear leg.*

Assailant at Your Side, Attacking with Overhead Swing

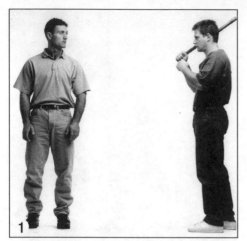

The assailant comes from the side.

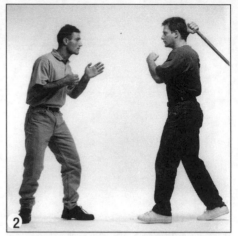

The assailant attacks with an overhead swing. Simultaneously execute a "stabbing" hand defense with a body turn that brings you in front of the assailant, and burst forward.

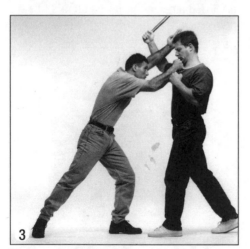

Execute the hand defense and initial counterattack. These actions, similar to the ones that follow, are executed as presented in the first technique of this chapter. It is important that your head be hidden under your arm.

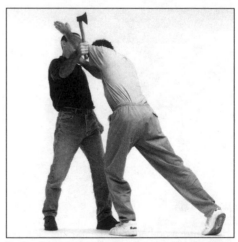

Defending an attack with an ax using the basic technique against an attack with a stick. This is an application of the technique *Overhead Swing – Stabbing Defense to the Inside of the Attack* against an attack with an ax.

Note: In this technique, it is important to execute the stabbing defense simultaneously with a body turn towards the assailant (you should not remain positioned sideways relative to the assailant) in order that the stick, when sliding along your forearm and arm, **will not hit your head**.

Overhead Swing – Stabbing Defense to the Outside of the Attack, Advancing with Two Steps

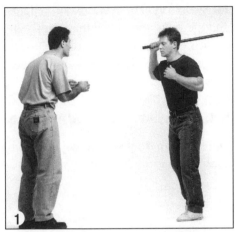

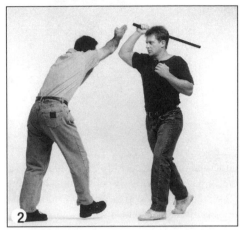

Starting position, i.e., a neutral stance.
Photograph 2: While bursting forward, execute a stabbing defense to the outside of the attacking forearm. The direction of the rapid advance is

diagonally forward, on the foot corresponding to the defending ("stabbing") hand (right foot, right hand), and crossing an imaginary line between you and the aggressor.

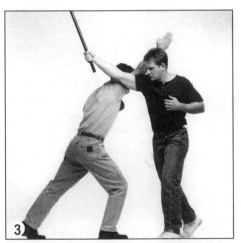

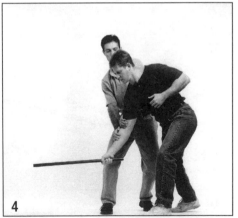

Completion of the defender's stabbing defense and his first step. While executing the "stab" your elbow faces down, your arm is straight, and the back of your hand faces out. (If necessary, you can counterattack from this position, without taking another step.)

Continue with an additional step on the foot opposite the defending ("stabbing") hand (left foot), so as to come almost behind the assailant. The purpose of this move is to reduce distance and serve as a preventive measure against any additional threats that may come from your right side or from the rear. Using one or both of your hands, and while advancing, pull the attacking hand down, restricting the assailant's ability to attack again.

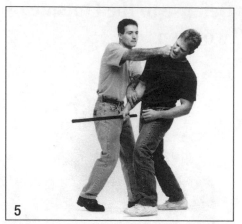

5

Grab and maintain control of the hand holding the stick, simultaneously delivering a counter-attack according to your position (alongside the assailant or behind him).

In this technique, you advance with **two steps**. The technique can be applied in different situations as follows:

1st situation: There are two assailants, and the regular defense may cause you to turn your back on, or come close to, the second one. The extra step is necessary here to avoid this problem. For further clarification, see Chapter 10: **Defense against Two Armed Assailants**.

Drawings 1a-1c illustrate what to do in such a situation.

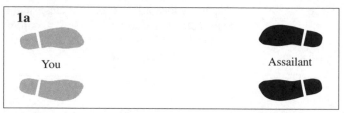

1a

You   Assailant

Drawing 1a: Situation in which you should go behind the aggressor.

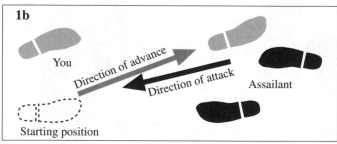

1b

You

Direction of advance

Direction of attack

Assailant

Starting position

Drawing 1b: Execute a forward burst with one step, simultaneously with a hand defense (as shown in photograph 3).

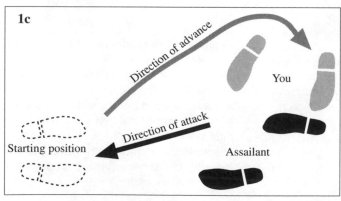

1c

Direction of advance

You

Direction of attack

Starting position

Assailant

Drawing 1c: With your second step, go behind the aggressor (as shown in photograph 4). In fact, the aggressor becomes a shield between you and the additional threat.

2nd situation: The aggressor comes from the side (or diagonally from the side) and delivers an overhead attack with the stick. Simultaneously with the stabbing defense, advance toward the assailant (on the same foot as the defending hand), turning your body to face him and shielding your head effectively with your arm. This will keep the stick from reaching your head. Drawings 2a and 2b illustrate how to apply this technique.

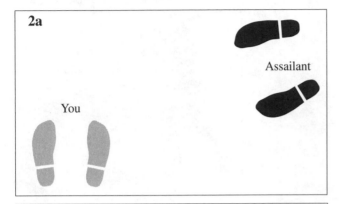

Drawing 2a: The aggressor is positioned diagonally to your right, preparing to attack you with an overhead swing.

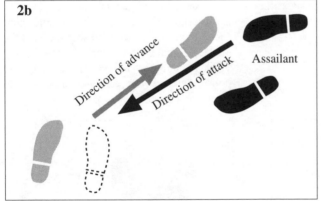

Drawing 2b: Perform a hand defense with your right hand while executing a body turn and advancing on your right foot.

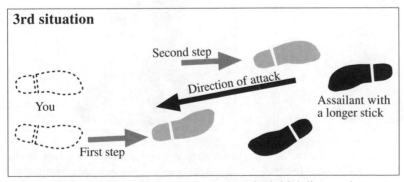

3rd situation: Against a longer stick or when the initial distance is greater, you will use **two steps**, since under these conditions advancing with a single step will not be sufficient.

Horizontal Swing from the Side – Bursting Forward (Baseball Bat Swing)

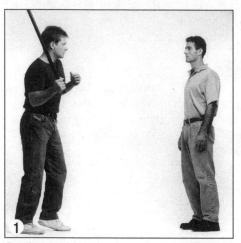

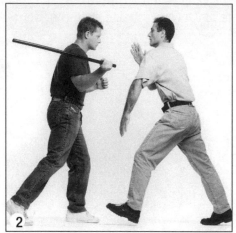

Starting position: for example, neutral stance.

The assailant advances while swinging his stick horizontally. Execute a body turn and burst forward, with your forward shoulder and leg on the side that is being attacked (the left side). While bursting forward, your front hand shall point down and your rear hand up, in order to shield your head.

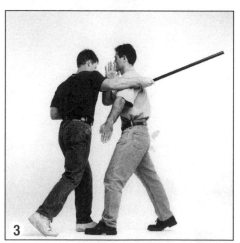

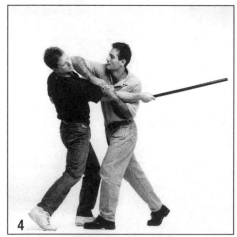

The moment of collision with the aggressor: your shoulder and arm come very close to the assailant's shoulder. The back of your lower hand and the palm of the other face outward.

Trap and lock the hand holding the stick, while executing a counterattack according to the distances involved (for example, a horizontal elbow strike to the assailant's head).

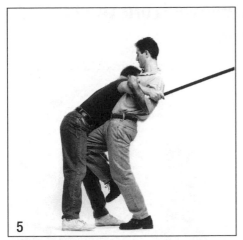

5

Further counterattack can be a knee kick to the assailant's groin.

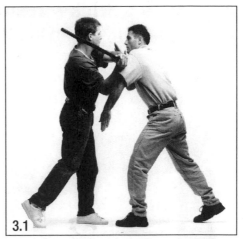

3.1

The same technique is performed against an attacker who holds the stick in both hands.

This defense is based almost exclusively on reducing the distance between you and the assailant. To achieve this goal, turn inward and burst straight forward, coming as close as possible to the aggressor, aiming your shoulder to reach the attacker's.

Note: The defender advances towards the shoulder of the attacker's arm which is swinging the stick.

The same steps shall be taken if the aggressor is striking while holding the stick in both hands (commonly referred to as a "baseball bat" swing), except that in this case you will collide with his upper arm (triceps) or forearm.

Start with a body defense that "pulls" you into a forward burst. Raise your rear hand quickly to the opposite cheek, while your front hand points down, with its outer, fleshy part facing out. (See photograph 3.1.)

If the stick does hit you, it will be with its least dangerous part, near where it is gripped, and it will impact a large area of your arm and back muscles, so that you suffer no real harm.

Possible variation: Burst forward, but in two steps. The first step is as previously demonstrated. The second, executed with the rear (right) foot in the direction of the stick's continuous movement, causes joined movement between you and the assailant, in a rotational motion. This movement reduces the impact with the attacker. However, the purpose of the rotation during the burst forward may also be to place the attacker between you and another aggressor (if there is such an aggressor behind you or to your left), or when you need to cover a longer distance in order to come closer to the attacker.

Stab with a Stick – Inside Defense from the Outside (Defending to the "Dead" Side)

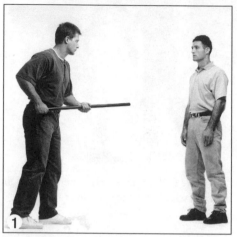

1

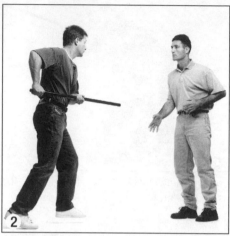

2

Starting position: for example, neutral stance. The aggressor is preparing to "stab" you with his stick.

The assailant advances, sending the stick forward in a stabbing movement. Start by executing an inside hand defense as your body follows with a forward lean and turn, shifting your weight diagonally forward and outward (to the right).

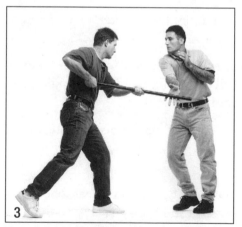

3

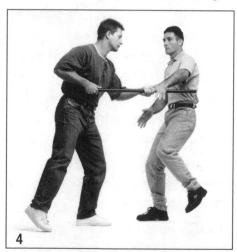

4

Execute an inside defense with your open hand, palm stretched. Lean slightly forward for greater reach, turn your body in an evasive action and burst diagonally forward. Your other (left) hand is brought near the opposite cheek.

Switch hands, while bursting diagonally forward. Your rear hand grabs the stick and your rear foot prepares to kick. The moment your forward leg touches the ground, your body is in position to deliver a kick.

Against a stab with a stick (or similar object such as sharp rod, pitchfork, or rifle with bayonet), execute an inside hand defense with your open, outstretched hand. For a wider defense, your palm is stretched so that your little finger is down and your thumb is up. Your body shall

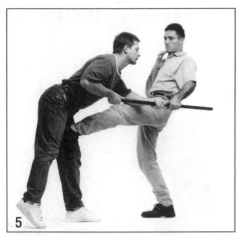

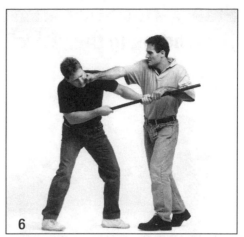

Grab the stick and kick the attacker in the groin; grabbing the stick is highly recommended in this situation, though it is not mandatory.

Further counterattack, for example, punching the attacker with your free hand.

lean forward and turn, to achieve an evasive movement and a longer reach that will enable you to deflect the stick at the beginning of the attack.

Note: If the weapon is indeed a spear, pitchfork, or bayoneted rifle, you must make sure that your hand **does not come into contact with the sharp (front) part of the weapon**. When deflecting the weapon, protect your other hand by moving it towards the opposite shoulder, out of the line of danger.

In some situations involving an attack with a relatively long weapon, as you deflect the weapon you can also pull it slightly with the defending hand in order to facilitate your forward advance. Your other hand replaces the deflecting hand, grabbing and pushing it (straightening the elbow) to overcome the recoil, and at the same time you kick the assailant in the groin.

Note: If the assailant is advancing quickly and forcefully, a kicking counterattack may not be suitable, since it requires a longer range. In this case, you can first attack by punch, elbow strike, knee, etc.

In integrating your moves, you must execute your kick with the proper timing. This will be accomplished with the kicking foot (left foot, see photograph 4), beginning its action a fraction of a second before the advancing foot (right foot) touches the ground. The advance in this case is therefore a sort of stomping or skipping step, performed diagonally forward. When the advancing foot hits the ground, its toes shall point slightly outward, giving the kicking leg an early start and greater range.

Variation: Deflect the weapon while sidestepping lightly and turning your body. Then quickly turn your body back, grabbing the weapon and delivering a regular kick to the assailant's groin.

Stab with a Stick – Inside Defense from the Inside (Defending to the "Live" Side)

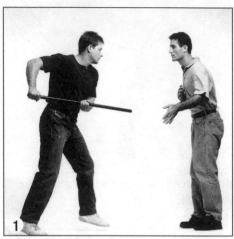

Starting position: for example, neutral stance. This version of the technique was originally intended for dealing with an attacker using a long bayoneted rifle. When the attacker starts his move, you start with your defense.

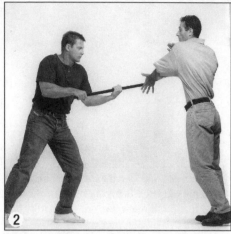

Execute an inside hand defense that "pulls" your upper body into a forward tilt while you perform a body turn, shifting your weight and bursting diagonally forward. The defending palm is open and stretched in order to extend its defending range.

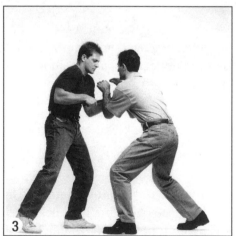

Bursting forward diagonally, bend your knees and lean slightly toward the weapon. To prevent the assailant from making further use of the weapon, by stabbing or by striking with the rear portion ("butt") of the stick, extend both your forearms forward and your elbows down to form a shield, keeping your elbows low and the palms of your hands facing the aggressor.

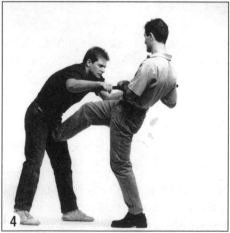

With your hands in a hook-like shape, grab the stick with a sweeping movement, lift it slightly, and with your rear leg execute a regular kick to the assailant's groin. Alternatively, you can kick him with your forward leg after advancing with a quick step.

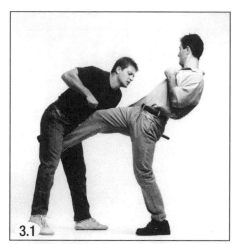

3.1

When there is no possibility for the assailant to strike you with the rear part of the weapon, counterattack in the same way as demonstrated in the previous technique, switching hands to grab the stick and delivering a regular kick with your rear foot.

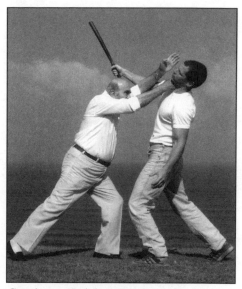

Grandmaster Imi demonstrating defense against an overhead swing.

This technique is performed especially when the attacker is using a weapon with a protruding rear part, such as a longer stick or a bayoneted rifle with a long butt.

Execute an inside defense while advancing towards the aggressor's "live" side. The hand defense and body defense are the same as in the previous technique, but once the stab is deflected, the assailant is liable to use the rear portion (butt) of the weapon in order to strike you.

Therefore, while advancing, lower your stance and send both forearms forward, while the inner (fleshy) part of the forearm, near your hand, slides down on the weapon. Then, grab the weapon and lift it so as to clear a path for a kick. Pulling the weapon also helps to control the aggressor and brings him closer to the kick.

The mirror image of the previous technique, *Defending to the "Dead" Side*, can also be used effectively to the live side, if the assailant has no possibility of attacking you with the rear part of the weapon for example, when he is holding the weapon at its very edge and no meaningful part of the stick protrudes behind his hand.

Neutralizing a Threat
at Gunpoint

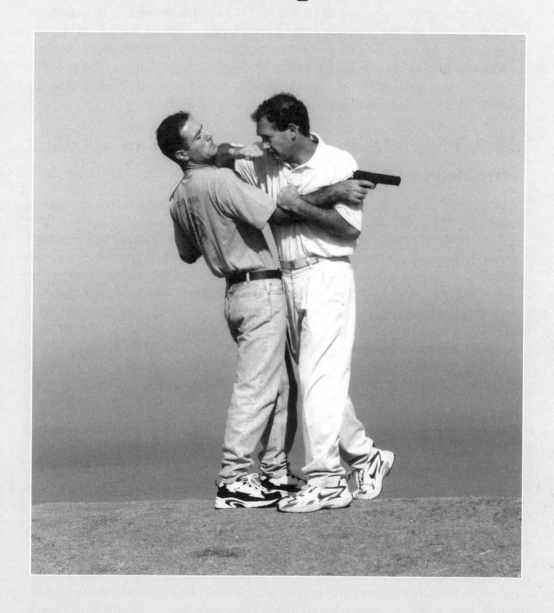

Chapter 4

Neutralizing a Threat at Gunpoint

When confronted by an assailant armed with a gun, **it is necessary to neutralize both the threat and the gunman**, using a fast, simple technique that is both safe and based on recognized principles and patterns of movement. This action is comprised of four components. (1) Defensive action: redirecting (hand defense) and avoiding (body defense) the line of fire. (2) Controlling the weapon. (3) Neutralizing the gunman by attacking him efficiently. (4) Disarming the gunman.

Basic Principles in Defending against an Assailant Threatening with a Handgun

Bear in mind that the person holding you at gunpoint probably **wants something from you**. This could be money, property, or information, or he may intend to take you as a hostage. In any case, **killing you is not usually his primary or immediate intent**. However, from the instant the threat exists, placing you and those nearby in danger, you have to act quickly and without hesitation! On the other hand, trying to overcome an armed gunman without having acquired adequate proficiency in the following techniques, is always **dangerous** and may ultimately result in severe injuries (or even death) to the defender as well as to those nearby. This delicate balance between attacking the gunman and refraining from such action should be **carefully considered** by anyone that becomes involved in an incident of this kind, weighing the relative risks that are inherent in each option.

Hint: The most opportune moment is when the aggressor's attention and focus are slightly distracted, such as when he is giving orders or having to answer a question addressed to him.

The direction in which the gun is pointed is termed the *"line of fire"* and is the line most dangerous to you and to other people nearby. Therefore, the first stage must be to **redirect the line of fire** by deflecting the gun and then maintaining control of it. As early as possible, move out of the line of danger and approach the aggressor from another angle, rendering it difficult for him to make further use of his gun.

Once you are no longer endangered by the gun itself, i.e., out of the line of fire, **the gunman himself becomes the main risk**. He must be rendered unable to make further use of the gun or attack you in any other way. Therefore, you now have to attack him with determination, for he (and not the gun) is now the immediate threat! After aggressively attacking the gunman, disarm him and end the incident by moving away, gun in hand.

Remember: The aggressor could be a trained combatant, and therefore **must not be underestimated**. Do not fix your eyes on the gun or "telegraph" your intention to take action against the aggressor. Clearly, it would be foolhardy, as well as a fundamental error, to count on any sort of "cooperation" from the assailant.

Act with determination against the assailant. Remember that the gunman, once engaged, will be fighting for his life, too!

You should gain control over the gun during the initial redirection of the line of fire. That control **must be maintained** until the weapon itself is removed from the gunman's hand. With one hand, grab the gun (or the hand holding it) with a firm grip, pressing hard to restrict movement. If you cannot do this, then grab the gun with both hands and kick the assailant hard.

Note: While disarming the assailant by rotating the gun in his palm, you should direct the movement of the barrel (the line of fire) to a higher or lower angle, in the event that there are bystanders near you. **By all means, make sure you do not redirect the line of fire back to yourself**. This principle is valid for all kinds of disarming: against threat of a handgun, rifle, shotgun, or submachine gun.

Caution: Due to the obvious risks involved in self-defense actions against a threat at gunpoint, these actions must never be performed solely on the basis of theoretical knowledge, **but only after extensive, repeated practice, under the supervision of an authorized instructor!**

Once you have learned the basic techniques and understood the underlying principles of action, practice the defenses at different ranges and angles and in different situations. **Examples**: neutralizing a threat when the aggressor is behind a barrier, neutralizing a threat while sitting in a car, neutralizing a threat when being shoved from behind or from the front, neutralizing a threat at close range, when you are lying down, etc.

Hint: It is important to perform the techniques while under self-imposed stress, in an attempt to simulate the danger under "realistic" conditions.

After disarming the aggressor, move away and proceed as required, i.e., keep him at a distance and in the line of fire until help arrives. A law-enforcement officer should maintain possession of the assailant's gun **but should also draw his own service weapon**, if there is time to do so. Remember, little is known about the exact state of the assailant's weapon. Is it serviceable? Is it loaded? Is it easy to operate? Sometimes, such as in the case with fighters in antiterrorist units, one will even have to shoot and injure the assailant immediately if he poses a genuine threat, especially in a situation where fighting continues and hostages are still in danger.

There are situations in which it will be difficult to apply the techniques against a handgun or a rifle threat. In such cases, **take no action unless you have no other chance of staying alive**, and the only possibility of survival is by taking action. Theoretically, since you are already considered dead (if a terrorist or a criminal is about to kill you), any action, even one involving a considerable risk, can only improve your chances to survive.

Types of Handguns – Brief Explanation

Primarily, there are two main types of handguns: **revolver** and **semi-automatic pistol**. When you deflect and grab a handgun, remember that **any pressure on the trigger is liable to cause the gun to go off**.

With most **semi-automatic** pistols, the slide (whose function is to load each new round) cannot move back while it is being held in place by the defender's hand. Therefore, if the aggressor pulls the trigger and the gun is ready for firing, a shot will most likely be fired, but the empty case will not be ejected. For the gun to be able to fire again, it must be reloaded manually (by drawing the slide back and releasing it).

In the case of a **revolver**, grabbing the body (and the cylinder) of the gun keeps the cylinder from turning, so that if the hammer is not cocked, a shot will not be fired. But if the hammer is cocked, pulling the trigger will fire a single bullet. In any event, a second shot will not be fired as long as the cylinder cannot rotate to place a live round in front of the hammer.

Remember: Whether in training or in an actual situation, the gun (even a toy pistol) has to be viewed as a **loaded, cocked weapon that can fire more than one bullet**! In training, you should unload and double-check any firearm (unless it is a dummy).

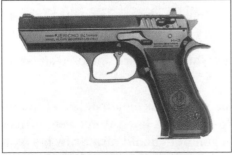

A semi-automatic pistol: Jericho 941.

The photograph of the Jericho was printed by courtesy of **Israel Military Industries** (**I.M.I.**).

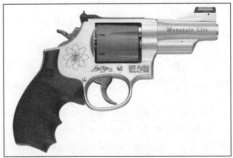

A revolver: 5 Shot .44 S&W Special Mountain Lite Revolver featuring Titanium cylinder and Aluminum Alloy frame. Courtesy of **Smith & Wesson, Springfield, Massachusetts**.

Threat from the Front, from a Distance

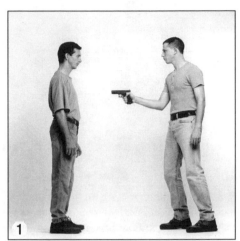

1

The assailant threatens you with a handgun, placed at a distance slightly beyond the reach of your outstretched arm. (In fact, this is the maximum possible distance for which you can utilize this defense.)

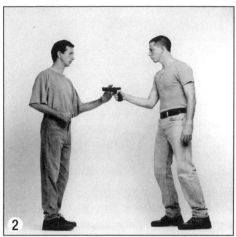

2

Send your hand directly alongside the pistol. The hand movement "pulls" your body into a turn, which enables you to reach the gun, and at the same time provides a body defense.

Note: Before sending out your hand to deflect the pistol, **be careful not to make any move that may reveal your intention to act**! Such a revealing movement, for example, could be shifting your weight forward at too early a stage, or leaning towards the weapon.

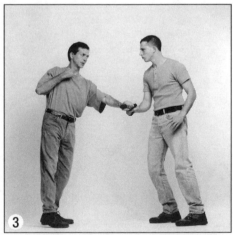

3

Rotate your palm, deflect the pistol sideways, and grab it, completing the body turn while shifting your weight forward. Grab the gun with your thumb down and fingers up, and straighten your elbow. Shift your weight diagonally forward, applying your weight to the pistol. As a result of the pressure, the gun is diverted and lowered.

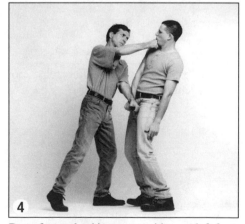

4

Burst forward, taking a step with your left foot, and deliver a punch to the assailant's chin or throat. The elbow of the arm that deflected the pistol is locked and straight. As a result, the pistol is now down and pointing to the side.

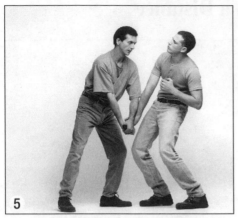

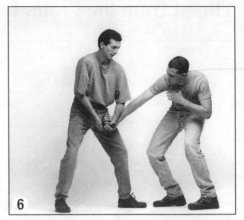

Move your rear (right) hand near your body so that it does not pass in front of the barrel of the gun (the line of fire), and grab the rear part of the gun, around the hammer.

Rotate the gun horizontally in the assailant's hand until it has moved $90°$ relative to its previous position. **Caution: Do not aim it at your own body!** This partly releases the gun from the grasp of the assailant, and also prevents his trigger finger from interfering with the disarming action.

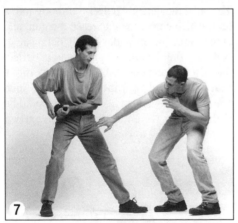

Pull the gun horizontally and forcefully from the assailant's hand and start moving back.

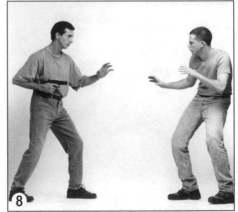

Possible conclusion of the incident: after moving away quickly, keep the assailant in the line of fire, at a suitable distance. Should the assailant pursue you, take appropriate action.

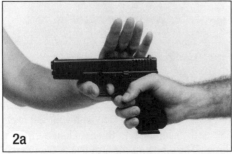

Close-up, photograph 2: The position of your palm at the initial point in time when you deflect the gun and start to grab it.

The gunman threatens you from the front, holding the pistol in one or both hands. The position of the gun ranges from zero distance (gun touching you) to about 8" (20 cm) from the end of your outstretched arm, i.e., an overall

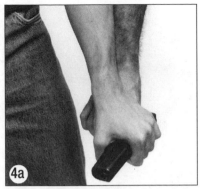

Close-up, photograph 4: Pressure on the gun, with straight elbow.

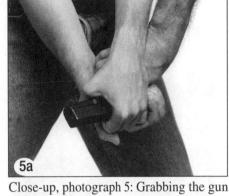

Close-up, photograph 5: Grabbing the gun with two hands.

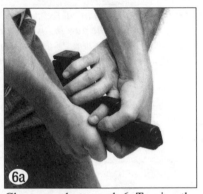

Close-up, photograph 6: Turning the pistol in the assailant's hand.

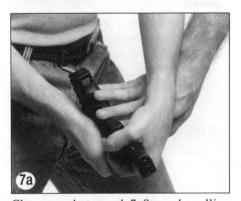

Close-up, photograph 7: Strongly pulling the gun and moving backward.

distance of some 30" (80 cm) from your body. The gun may be held at different heights, anywhere from the stomach to the head. It should be emphasized that **the gun is to be deflected in a straight line to the side**, and not diagonally up or down. This is to ensure that the gun is moved off your body in the shortest line possible. When grabbing the pistol, your thumb shall point down and your fingers up.

Grabbing the gun correctly will usually prevent the trigger from being pulled, but this is a side effect, not essential to the success of the technique. When you are shifting your weight forward and straightening your elbow, apply your weight in such a way that will severely limit the movement of the assailant's hand holding the gun. The pistol is brought near the assailant's body and in front of your rear leg, with the barrel pointing sideways, such that any attempt by the gunman to pull the gun and aim it at you will fail.

The technique used in variation 3 (V3) against a close threat to the stomach is basically identical to our initial technique. The body defense is very important here. You should take care not to allow the gun to get caught in your clothing, which

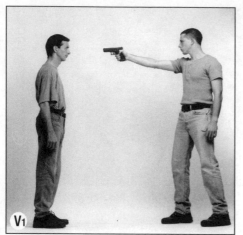

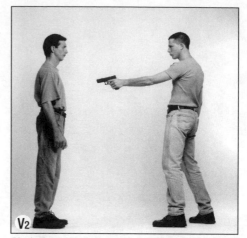

*Variation: **The aggressor points the gun at your head**. Essentially, execute an identical technique. The moment you start raising your hand to grab the gun, you should also move your head sideways, away from the line of fire.*

*Variation: Execute an identical technique, with the assailant **holding the gun in his left hand** and standing in front of you. In this situation you can also perform the technique in mirror image, i.e., deflect and grab the pistol with your right hand, burst forward on your right leg, and counterattack with your left hand. You could also use the variation demonstrated in the next technique.*

would restrict the defensive movement of the hand. To prevent this, pull your stomach in slightly. Another effective defense that can be used in this situation resembles the defense against a hand-gun: ***Threat from the Side, in Front of Your Arm***. (See later in this chapter.) That technique is best suited in the event that the gun is held very low.

Stages of Learning

A. Practice moving your hand quickly to the height of the pistol, without turning your body.

B. Practice Stage A, followed by a body turn and a deflection while grabbing the pistol. Refrain from any "telegraphing" of your moves.

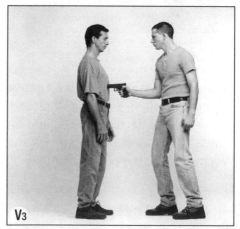

*Variation: You are being threatened at gunpoint, from the front, **with the pistol either touching you or very close to you**. You should perform a technique identical to the one performed against a threat at long range.*

C. From this point on, use the usual method of learning. Break the technique down into stages, and then combine them into a flowing movement.

Diagonal Threat from the Front, from a Distance – Entry on "Live" Side

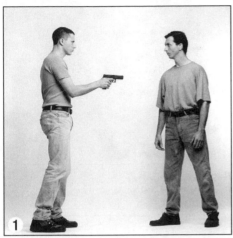

The aggressor stands diagonally in front of you. The direction of threat matches the hand holding the gun. (The assailant holds the gun in his right hand and is standing at your right.)

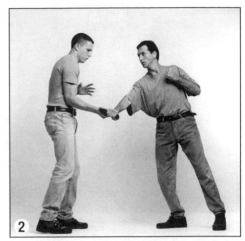

Deflect the pistol in the usual way, with the hand closer to the gun. Contrary to the previous technique, this action will not bring the gun closer to the assailant's body.

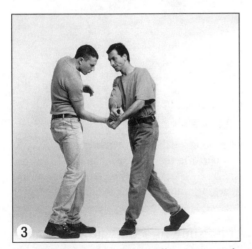

If you feel that you are standing at an angle that does not allow you to advance to striking range and therefore you cannot control the gun effectively, then you should grab the gun with both hands, securing it, and advance with a bursting step on your rear leg, so that you will be able to kick the gunman.

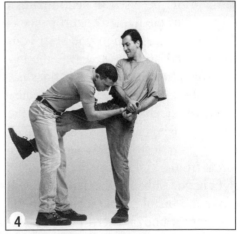

Deliver a regular kick to the assailant's groin with your forward (right) leg. Hit with your instep, shin, or knee, according to the distance between you and the gunman. At this stage, you can start disarming the assailant by rotating the gun in his hand.

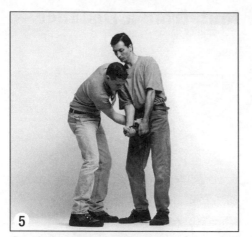

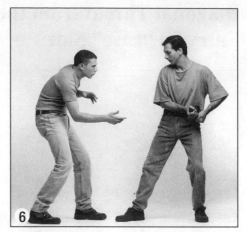

Conclude disarming the assailant by rotating the gun. The barrel is directed to the side during the entire period of engagement.

Retreat backwards.

When the gunman is standing diagonally in front of you, you must apply the basic technique according to the same principles used in neutralizing a threat from the front. The difference is that in this case, when you shift your weight and advance towards the aggressor (photograph 2). This does not place the gun closer to him as occurs when you neutralize the threat with the hand opposite that of the assailant, i.e., using your left hand to neutralize a threat from a gun held in the assailant's right hand. Although the deflection will move the pistol further away from the

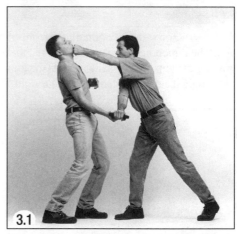

Depending on the situation, in many cases you can perform the regular technique in mirror image, by advancing with your right foot and attacking with your left hand. Force the barrel sideways, straightening your elbow.

assailant's body rather than closer to it, after bursting forward you will usually achieve a range suitable for the hand attack. (See photograph 3.1.) However, since you may still find yourself beyond striking range, you must grab the gun with two hands as described, advance and attack the assailant by kicking him in the groin. This will ultimately solve the problem of distance.

In many cases, you will be able to improve your position and achieve a situation in which you are standing face-to-face with the threat, enabling "regular" execution of the technique. This clearly requires time, as well as the possibility for such action.

Note: If the assailant is holding his weapon in both hands, you can basically apply the same technique used against a one-handed grip hold. However, such a situation may call for minor adjustments on the part of defender, such as enhancing your grip with both your hands and kicking the gunman in the groin instead of delivering a punch to his head.

When Should You Apply the Technique Using Your "Other" Hand?

- If there is another person, located on your right, you will have to deflect the weapon to your left side, using your right hand, so as **not to place this person in the line of fire**. Otherwise he may be shot as a result of the gun going off.

- As shown above in the previous technique (photograph 1), a situation may arise when the gunman is standing at a distance, either to your right or diagonally in front of you. In such a circumstance, you may be forced to shift your weight onto the foot that is closer to the aggressor in order to reach the gun. This may render it harder to apply the regular technique, by bursting forward and shifting your weight onto the gun. Here, grabbing the gun with both hands will be an effective option for gaining better control of the gun. Executing a kick will then serve as the initial counterattack in this case.

- When the gun is in front of you, held to the left of the center of your body, use your right hand to deflect the threat so that the gun moves off the target, covering the shortest possible distance.

- When the movement of your left hand is restricted, e.g., the assailant is grabbing your left hand or arm and thus preventing it from executing the defense, or when your left hand has been injured.

A Real-Life Story

Samuel Lichtenfeld, the celebrated father of Grandmaster Imi Sde-Or (Lichtenfeld), was Chief Detective of the police department in Bratislava, Slovakia. Due to his activities he would occasionally hide his personal weapon, a revolver, in one of the closets at home.

One day, Imi's elder brother found the gun and began playing with it. Totally unaware of the danger, he aimed the gun at Imi's head at close range and pulled the trigger. Imi, who was only 13 at the time, instinctively struck the gun and deflected it. As result , the bullet went straight into the wall, and Imi was not even scratched.

Threat from Behind, at Close Range

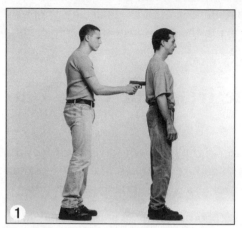

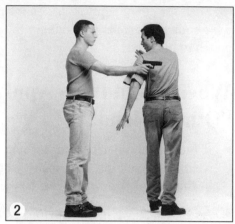

The aggressor threatens from behind, with a pistol at your back.

Photograph 2: Look behind you to see what is happening, i.e., which hand is holding the gun and where his other hand is. This move is

a completely natural reaction towards one who has initiated verbal or physical contact with you from behind. Deflect the attacker's forearm or his pistol. This leads you into a body turn and a forward burst towards the gunman.

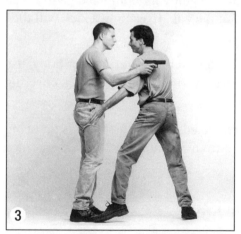

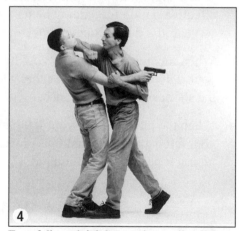

After deflecting the gun, move your deflecting hand diagonally forward and out, sliding along the inside of the attacker's arm. Burst towards the assailant. Your forward leg is on the same side as the defending hand.

Forcefully and tightly trap the assailant's forearm between your upper arm, forearm, hand, and chest, and at the same time strike his jaw or throat with a horizontal elbow punch forward and inward.

In this technique we observe the following four basic components: (1) Neutralizing the threat of the handgun by redirecting the line of fire away from your body. This, combined with a body defense, creates the earliest overall defense. (2) Grabbing the hand holding gun, to eliminate any further use. (3) Attacking and overcoming the gunman. (4) Disarming the assailant.

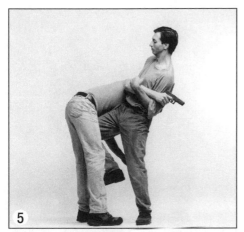

Grab the gunman's shoulder and deliver a knee to his groin. The gun may fall from the attacker's hand at this stage or may have already fallen during the previous one.

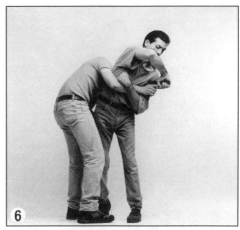

Should the pistol still be in the assailant's hand, execute a sharp body turn in order to see if it is there and reach for the gun quickly. Grab the gun, with the palm of your hand facing down (thumb directed towards you).

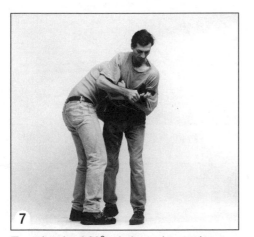

Turn the pistol 90° relative to its previous position. **Caution**: Do not ever direct the barrel towards your body!

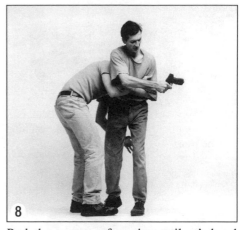

Push the gun away from the assailant's hand in the direction of his index finger. (See close-ups 6a, 6b, 7a, and 8a.)

It is extremely important to take a good look before committing yourself to any defensive action. You will need to see whether the position of the gun or the gunman will make it difficult to apply the technique, e.g., if the gun is too far away or too close, or if the assailant's other hand (the one not holding the pistol) is touching you, and not the gun itself. After deflecting the gun, move towards the assailant, sliding your deflecting hand parallel to the gunman's arm, and securing his forearm. This is done in order to keep the assailant from pulling the gun back and redirecting it at you. The first counterattack you can execute is a horizontal

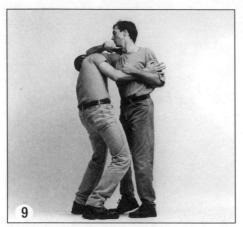

While moving away from the aggressor, you can launch another attack, e.g., hit him with the barrel of the gun or deliver a horizontal elbow strike.

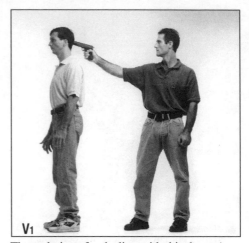

The technique for dealing with this threat (gun pointed at your head from behind) is almost identical to the previous one, when the threat was to your back.

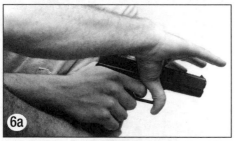

Close-up, photograph 6: Body turn, reaching for the gun.

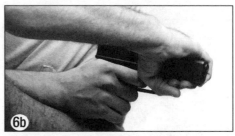

Close-up, photograph 6: Grabbing the gun.

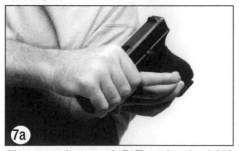

Close-up, photograph 7: Turn the pistol 90° relative to the assailant's hand.

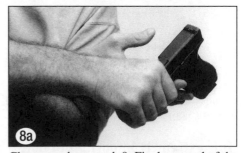

Close-up, photograph 8: Final removal of the pistol, pushing it away from the gunman's hand.

elbow strike inward, accompanied by a forward movement (if dictated by the distance between you and the adversary). If the gunman is too far from you and you cannot reach him with an elbow strike, a straight punch can be delivered instead. Then you may continue to close the distance between you and the assailant, delivering elbow strikes as needed.

You can execute the deflection and the body turn either to the right or to the left, whichever way you feel most comfortable, but also depending upon the specific circumstances. Of course, the technique is identical whether you turn to your right or to your left. (See section at the end of the previous technique: *When Should You Apply the Technique Using Your "Other" Hand?*)

The technique will be basically the same when the pistol is held at your head from behind (as shown in photograph V₁). However, in this case it is essential that you move your head as soon as possible towards the gunman's head, with a quick turning motion of the head accompanied by a body turn, while bursting towards the gunman. (See: *Threat to the Head from the Side – Turning*.) The main difference is that here you move the target (i.e.: your head) **before** deflecting the hand holding the gun.

Threat from the Side, Behind Your Arm

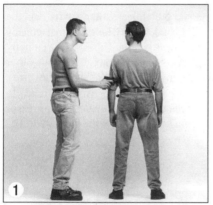

1

The assailant places the pistol at your side, behind your arm.

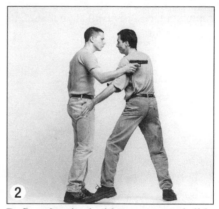

2

Deflect the pistol with your arm and slide it alongside the attacker's arm. At the same time, turn your body towards the assailant and advance with a quick burst forward in his direction.

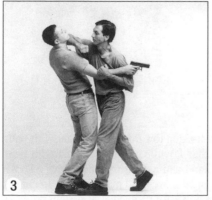

3

Secure (trap) the assailant's forearm and deliver an elbow strike to his chin or throat. Continue exactly as in the previous technique.

Execute the turn towards the gunman, moving **in the fastest and shortest way possible**. In the situation shown, turn to the left (counterclockwise). In effect, this is almost identical to the technique of neutralizing a threat from behind at close range, except for the relative positions of the attacker and the defender. Obviously, performing this technique you need a smaller body turn in order to face the assailant.

Threat from the Side, in Front of Your Arm

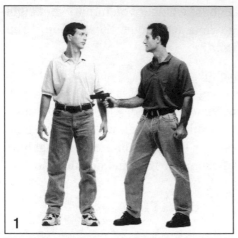

1

The gunman places the pistol at your side, in front of your arm.

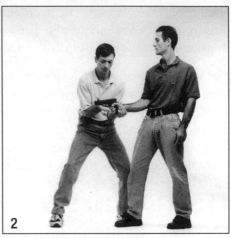

2

Deflect and grab the assailant's wrist and the back of his hand, while taking a step diagonally back and towards him. This serves as a body defense. At the same time, raise your other hand (keeping it well out of the line of fire), so that it is parallel to the pistol and ready to grab it. This will also prevent the aggressor from turning and pointing the gun at you.

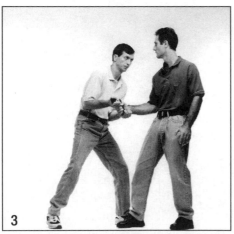

3

As soon as possible, grab the barrel of the gun firmly with your right hand and start breaking the aggressor's hold on the gun.

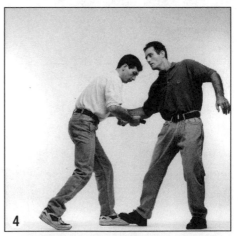

4

Push the gun towards the assailant with your right hand, while pulling his wrist with your left hand and executing a body turn. These combined moves will make your action much more powerful. If needed, it is now possible to retreat from the vicinity of the assailant.

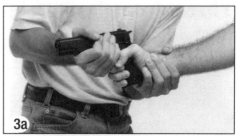

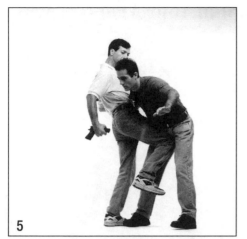

Close-up, photograph 3: Grabbing the gun and the hand holding it.

5

Continue with a knee to the aggressor's groin. You may now also add further counterattacks. Immediately move away from the disarmed assailant, stepping back with your right foot, followed by steps with the left and then the right foot again.

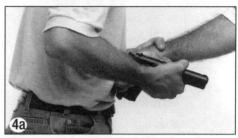

Close-up, photograph 4: Turning the gun forcefully inside the hand holding it, to disarm the assailant. The barrel should be parallel to the underside of the gunman's forearm, and turned horizontally.

When you deflect the gun, pull in your stomach and quickly move diagonally backwards toward the gunman, moving out of danger. Deflect the threatening hand near the wrist and the back of the hand, in order to stabilize and prevent the wrist from bending during the defense.

Caution: If the assailant's wrist bends, it may cause the line of fire to be directed back to you.

While deflecting the gun with one hand, bring your other hand alongside the pistol as quickly as possible, but **without moving it in front of the barrel**. In effect, both hands perform the same movement simultaneously: the deflecting hand moves the gun forward while the other hand, in an almost identical motion, comes alongside the gun. Position your elbows virtually in front of your ribs.

Once you have disarmed the gunman, you can move away or alternatively, proceed with several powerful counterattacks as required (a punch, a strike with the weapon, or a kick), and only then move a safe distance away.

If the aggressor is on your other side (i.e., threatening with the right hand from the right side), the approach will be made towards his live side. (See next technique.)

Threat from the Side, in Front of Your Arm – Moving to the Gunman's "Live" Side

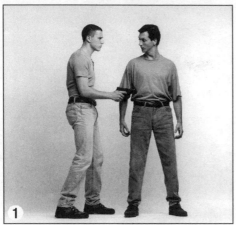

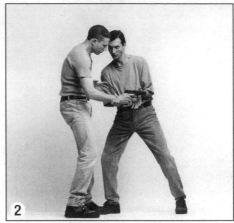

The gunman is threatening you from the side while the handgun is in front of your arm. You will move towards the aggressor's live side.
Photograph 2: As in the previous technique, *Threat from the Side, in Front of Your Arm*,

here too, you deflect the pistol (grabbing the gunman's wrist and palm) and move diagonally back and towards the aggressor. Simultaneously, and with the same motion, bring your other hand alongside the gun in order to grab it.

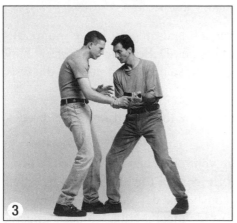

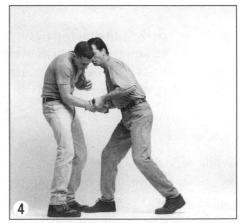

Grab the barrel with your far hand and start applying leverage to the gun.

You will break the assailant's grip on the pistol by applying leverage to it. Rotate the gun 90° relative to its previous position, while your whole body pivots to help with the motion.

In principle, this technique is identical to *Threat from the Side, in Front of Your Arm*, except that this time you move to the live side of the assailant. Disarming is also different. You need to disarm the gunman in two stages as follows: First, turn the barrel of the gun in the direction of the back of the hand holding it, and then pull it out of his hand.

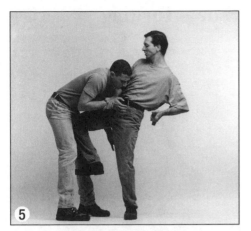

5

Pull the gun out of the assailant's hand while advancing with your rear leg, in order to deliver a knee to his groin. Counterattack and then continue by moving a safe distance away. You may also execute additional attacks before or while you withdraw.

Remember: Although you have successfully disarmed your opponent, you should **counterattack immediately**, before the gunman has time to recover. If you do not move fast enough and as long as you remain near him on his live side, you will be making it easier for him to attack first.

Your first counterattack is performed with a kick, as both your hands are occupied. Based on the distance and angle, you may kick with either leg.

Variation: Perform the same technique but from the opposite side, i.e., with the gunman at your left, holding the gun in his left hand.

It is extremely important to practice neutralizing threats from different angles and in different situations. Clearly, you should not become accustomed to applying this technique only in the situation most comfortable to you!

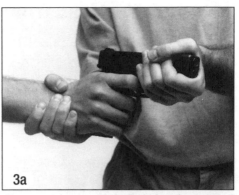

3a

Close-up, photograph 3: Grabbing the gun and the assailant's hand or wrist.

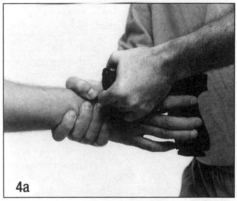

4a

Close-up, photograph 4: Breaking the hold and rotating the gun with a strong leverage action.

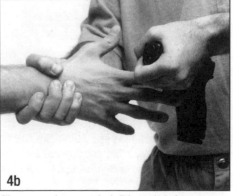

4b

Close-up, photograph 4: Disarming the gunman by pulling the gun away.

Threat to the Head from the Side – Turning

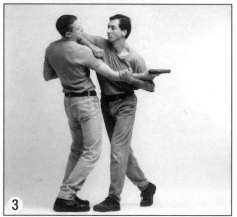

1

The assailant places the handgun alongside, or behind your head, level with your ear. (See diagram below.)

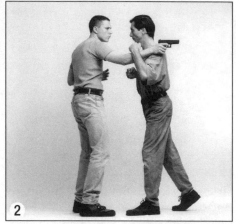

2

Turn your head and body simultaneously towards the gunman, and advance rapidly towards him. This removes you from the "line of fire" to an area behind the gun. At the same time, raise your hand in a hook form, around the assailant's forearm, and pull it slightly sideways.

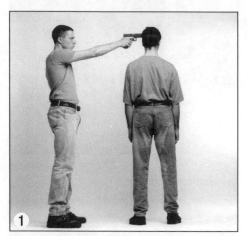

3

Pull the assailant's forearm down, grab it, and counterattack. Do not permit his arm to become stuck on top of your shoulder but bring it down to your chest level. This will provide greater distance between the gun, which can still be fired, and your head (or ear). Proceed as in the technique *Threat from Behind, at Close Range.*

This technique is based on ***Threat from Behind, at Close Range***. Here, the emphasis of the technique, and specifically in its leading movement, should be on the simultaneous and sudden turning of your head and body towards the aggressor and rapidly advancing towards him. This will take you out of danger. The same will be done when a gun is aimed at your head from the rear. The function of the near hand is to easily trap the forearm and control the hand holding the pistol, in order to deflect and lower it to chest level.

Drawing: If the gun is aimed at area A, this technique (turning) should be preferred. If the gun is pointed at area B (the "front half"), the following technique should then be preferred.

The counterattacks and disarming are as described in the technique ***Threat from Behind, at Close Range***. The distance for counterattacking is usually suitable for an elbow strike, but if the distance is greater, it may be necessary to use a straight punch as the initial attack.

Threat to the Head, from the Side – Deflecting and Grabbing the Gun

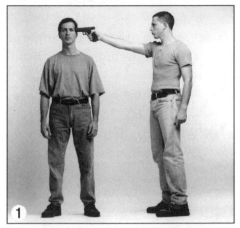

The gunman places the handgun at or very near the side of your head (from the ear and forward, i.e., the *"front half"*).

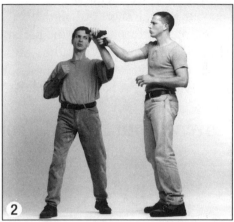

Grab the pistol, send it down in the direction of the assailant, and counterattack. All this is accomplished in precisely the same manner as described in the first technique: ***Threat from the Front, from a Distance***.

Move your head back and towards the gunman, so as to move out of the line of fire. Simultaneously with the head movement, raise your hand quickly and bring it alongside the pistol in order to deflect and grab it. At the same time, advance towards the assailant with a diagonal step to the side and slightly backwards.

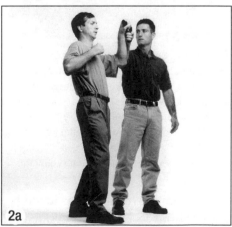

Stage 2, pictured from the defender's side.

This technique is basically identical to that used in ***Threat from the Front, from a Distance***. Two actions, a head movement and a hand movement, are performed simultaneously in order to create the earliest possible defense. When the gun is pushed against your head, you should turn your head slightly (body defense) in the opposite direction, away from the gunman, to make the weapon slide away from your head. From the aspect of timing, your head moves out of danger even before your hand reaches the gun.

This technique, once learned, can be applied in the following situations: against threat from a pistol at the side of the head; when the assailant is directly or diagonally opposite you; at short or long range; and others. Sometimes this technique will be preferable, and sometimes the previous one is better, depending on **the angle at which the aggressor is standing and the exact location of the gun at your head**. For example, this technique is preferable if the pistol is pointed at your temple, and the previous one is better if the gun is behind or above your ear.

Threat from Behind, from a Distance

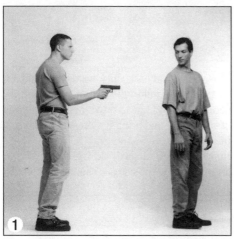 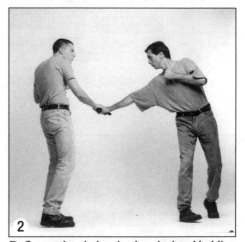

The attacker threatens with the handgun directly or diagonally behind you, from a distance. For executing this technique, the most suitable distance between the gun and your back is 15"-25" (40-65 cm). Look casually behind you to judge the distance from the gun, but without lingering on it. The defense should be executed immediately after this preliminary glance.

Deflect and grab the pistol or the hand holding it. This deflecting movement of your hand leads into the rest of your actions: a body turn that will get you away from the line of fire, and a bursting step towards the adversary. Shift your weight onto the gun and press on it, downward and towards the aggressor.

This technique requires considerable practice, since it involves a **greater risk** than the previous techniques described in this chapter. The problem in this case is that

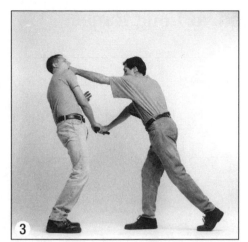

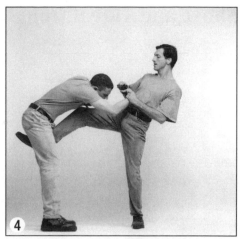

Burst towards the gunman on your right leg (the same side as the deflecting hand), and counterattack decisively with a straight punch. Note to stay away from the initial line of fire.

With the gun barrel **pointing sideways**, use your other hand to grab the assailant's wrist, and counterattack again by kicking or kneeing him in the groin. Use whichever leg is more convenient (in the photograph, the defender is advancing with the rear leg and kicking with his front) and then disarm the assailant, rotating the gun in his hand.

when you are looking behind you, you can see the gun with only one eye. Since this does not allow for a three-dimensional view, the distance cannot be judged accurately! Therefore, this technique should be applied **only when there is no other alternative**, i.e., only in life-or-death situations. In training, emphasis is placed on correctly estimating the distance, deflecting the gun while moving the body out of the line of fire, and exercising precision while grabbing the gun.

Note: If the assailant is situated diagonally behind you, neutralize the threat by using essentially the same technique. In most cases you will be able to see the gun with both eyes and judge the distance correctly.

The principles in this technique are as those used in neutralizing a *Threat from the Front, from a Distance*. Beginning with a hand movement that will "propel" the body into a body defense (to get out of the line of fire), grab the gun as you advance and shift your weight towards the assailant and down onto the gun. Execute hand or leg attacks according to the range you have achieved. Finally, disarm the gunman.

Shove and Threat from Behind, at Long Range

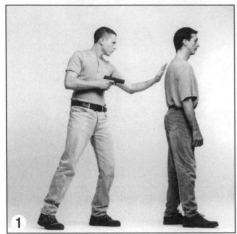

The technique presented here is appropriate in a situation where the gunman's free hand is extended forward and the gun is far from your back. The gunman may be standing in a stationary position, he may be pushing you, applying constant pressure, or, as shown, he may be delivering bursting shoves, forcing you forward. The assailant shoves you and points his gun at you. You have already managed to look back and assess the situation.

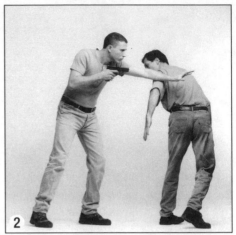

Evade the shove by sidestepping slightly and pivoting on one foot in order to move out of the line of danger. The turn is **to the outside of the shoving hand** (not to the hand holding the gun). In this stage the pivoting leg is the front one.

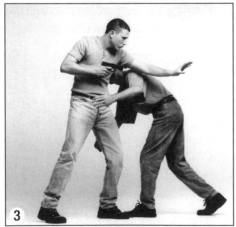

The assailant will continue to move forward as you approach him from the side. The side-stepping (left) foot should be the rear one, and the body should turn in its direction, e.g., to the left, as shown in the photograph.

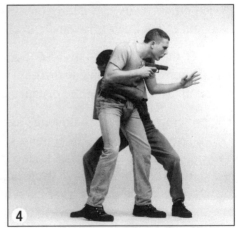

Pivot on your front (left) leg and grab the attacker's stomach and groin, with your knees bent, your back straight, and your stomach and chest pressed against him. You can also grab the forearm of the hand holding the gun.

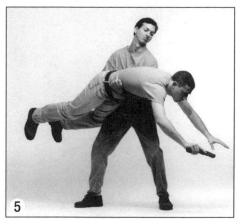

5

Lift the assailant with your forearm at his groin, pull him back with your lower hand and push his upper body with yours.

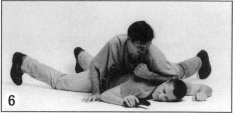

6

Throw your legs back and fall hard on the aggressor, forming an "X", with your chest on the center of the assailant's back. Before hitting the ground, move your hands out from under the assailant's body, and counterattack as early as possible.

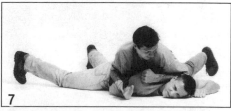

7

Possible counterattack: elbow strike to the back of the neck or punch to the temple. Then get hold of the gun and disarm the assailant.

This technique is appropriate both against a static threat or a push with constant pressure, and also against bursting shoves, which are more serious and dangerous. The technique demands precise timing and a very high degree of skill! Perform it after you have discerned the speed and timing of the aggressor's leading shoves. It is imperative that you spin around **at the precise moment that the assailant intends to shove**, so that he encounters an empty space, which will adversely affect his balance. Do not apply this technique after having been shoved, but always **before** the first or next shove! Turn your body towards the pivoting foot. Begin the turn when the pivoting foot is to the rear. If you turn to the left, you should pivot on the left (rear) foot, pushing strongly with your right (forward) leg.

Emphases for practice: (1) Evading the line of threat. (2) With a straight back, grabbing the assailant's body and groin (effective for neutralizing him). (3) Falling on the aggressor with great force, sufficient to stun him. In the fourth stage, it is also optional to grab the assailant's forearm (the hand holding the gun).

Alternative techniques:

- If conditions permit, especially if the gun is not too far away from you, you can also apply the previous technique: *Threat from Behind, from a Distance*.

- If the assailant shoves you with his gun dug into your back, apply the regular technique: *Threat from Behind, at Close Range*.

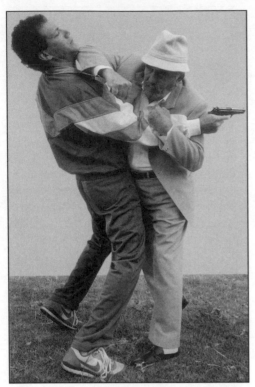

Gramdmaster Imi Sde-Or demonstrating defense against a gun threat from behind.

A Real-Life Story

Joseph had been training in Krav Maga for several years. At one stage in his life he worked as a salesman in a gunshop selling small arms (mainly handguns). One day one of his workmates took a gun from the store, loaded it with a full magazine, cocked it, and then removed the magazine. Joseph warned him that the gun was probably loaded, that there could still be a round left in it. His friend insisted that the gun was empty, and an argument ensued, during which he jokingly aimed the gun at the center of Joseph's body, intending to pull the trigger and thereby prove that the gun was indeed empty. Joseph preformed the technique he had learned in Krav Maga, deflecting the gun; and when it went off, the bullet hit the counter.

Neutralizing a Threat of Rifle, Shotgun or Submachine Gun

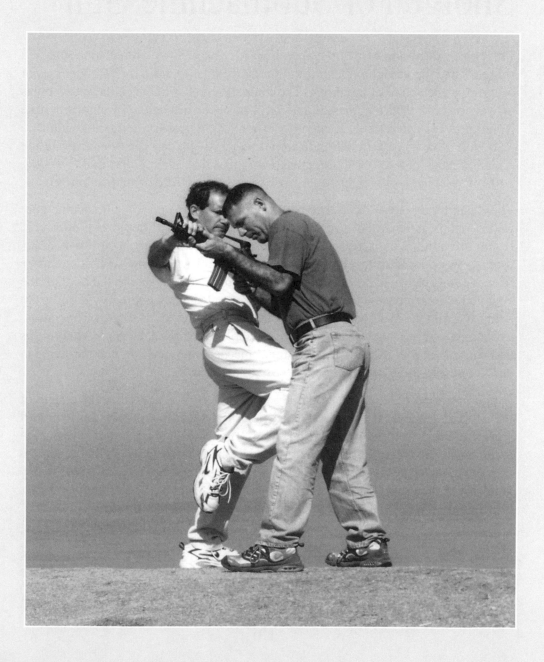

Chapter 5

Neutralizing a Threat of Rifle, Shotgun or Submachine Gun

There are many similarities between the rifle (as well as submachine gun and shotgun) and the handgun. The most important similarity, from the defender's point of view, is the nature of the threat. The main differences between these two types of weapons are their lengths and the ways that they are held. If we consider the techniques for neutralizing a threat from a handgun and for defending against a stab with a stick or a rifle with a bayonet attached, we can combine some of the common principles to create effective techniques that are appropriate for dealing with an assailant posing a threat (at close range) with a rifle or submachine gun.

There is a fundamental difference between the handgun and the submachine gun; aside from the difference in size and how they are held, they differ in their operation. If you are holding the submachine gun's barrel, the assailant can still fire all his rounds, as opposed to the semi-automatic handgun where only one shot can be fired when someone is holding the barrel and slide. This is due to the hold on the slide, which prevents the handgun from being loaded again and a new round from being fed into the chamber. With a revolver, depending on its mode of operation, as long as you hold the cylinder, only one shot can be fired, at most. Many rifles and shotguns are equipped with a manual mechanism, meaning that the gunman has to **operate them manually** in order to reload and fire the next shot.

Exactly as in neutralizing a handgun threat, you must first neutralize the danger of the immediate threat, i.e., **redirect the line of fire by deflecting the firearm and simultaneously removing your body from that line**. You must then prevent the assailant from making further use of the weapon and restrict his (or her) freedom of movement, and especially that of the weapon. Simultaneously (or immediately afterwards), you should neutralize the assailant with an appropriate counterattack. Finally, you must also disarm him and distance yourself from the danger zone.

Note: As a result of the lethal nature of the firearms dealt with in this chapter, a maximum degree of caution is required when utilizing the following techniques. This is obviously a matter for experts who are totally proficient in this domain. (See also the relevant warning in the previous chapter: **Neutralizing a Threat at Gunpoint**.)

Principles for the techniques presented in this chapter:

- **The best time for the neutralizing action is the moment that the assailant's attention is not focused completely on you or on his weapon**. For example: when the attacker is behind you, you can turn to look at him and plead with him, ask a question, or just speak. This allows you to check the possibility of executing a suitable technique while distracting the assailant's attention. It is common that during the commission of street crimes, the victim often has some face-to-face conversation with the assailant. When possible, make use of this fact.

- **Deflect the barrel of the gun in the fastest and shortest way possible**. Very often, the situation and the way you are standing mandate that you deflect the barrel of the gun with your right hand, at other times with your left hand. Sometimes, you might even find yourself in a situation where you can **choose** which hand to use for this action.

- It may sometimes be imperative to deflect the gun in the direction that is less convenient for you, so as **not to redirect the line of fire towards innocent people** standing near you.

- **Deflect the gun and burst towards the assailant**, coming close to him. This will make it extremely difficult for him to operate the weapon against you.

- The techniques for neutralizing a threat from an assailant holding a short rifle or a submachine gun **in one hand**, are basically similar to that used for neutralizing a handgun threat.

- When the assailant is holding the rifle or submachine gun **in both hands**, it will be much more difficult for you to move the gun, and even harder to maintain control over it once you have deflected it in a particular direction. Therefore, even more than when neutralizing a threat from a handgun, you will have to rely here on creating a body defense by moving in, immediately following your initial deflection of the gun. **This will keep you out of the line of fire**.

- **Hitting the assailant** will enable you to remove the gun from his hands more freely. Actions that are based more on **rotating** the gun rather than on **pulling** it, will make it easier for you to take it away from the assailant.

The following techniques are concerned with neutralizing the threat of a rifle, shotgun or submachine gun, when the assailant is either in front of you or behind you. Once you thoroughly understand these techniques (and those for neutralizing a handgun threat), you should practice neutralizing threat of a rifle or submachine gun from different directions, distances, and angles. Then you will also train in various positions and situations, e.g., while you are standing or sitting, and when the assailant is shoving, pulling, or grabbing you, etc.

Threat from the Front – Weapon Held in One Hand

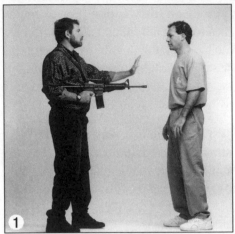

The assailant threatens you with an assault rifle (or submachine gun) that he holds in one hand. The range from your body to the weapon makes it possible to deflect and grab it.

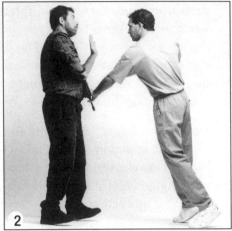

Similar to the basic technique against handgun threat, start with the hand action, add the body turn and, shifting your weight diagonally forward, deflect the gun to the side and grab it where it can be easily held, while applying pressure diagonally downwards.

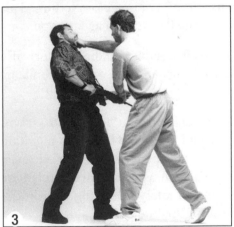

Burst forward (on the same foot as the deflecting hand) while applying pressure (sideways and downwards) on the gun, and counterattack. According to the way the attacker is holding the gun, you can pull it slightly (with a straight elbow) in order to assist your forward advance.

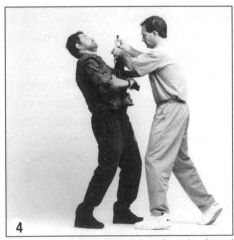

Grab the barrel with both hands, raise it and send it towards the assailant's head.

This technique is, in effect, identical in action and principle to the basic technique for neutralizing handgun threat from the front. Such action can be taken mainly when the assailant is holding the weapon in one hand or at very close range, and if it is at all possible to grab the forward part of the gun, that is, if it is not too short or broad and if the assailant's forward hand does not hinder this action.

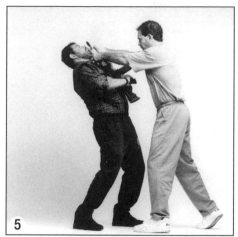

5

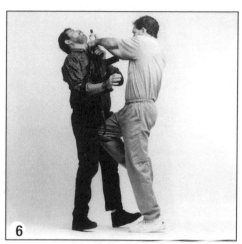

6

Using the gun or with your fists, strike the assailant's head.

Photograph 6: Attack again, e.g., with a knee kick to the assailant's groin. In order to disarm

him, shift one hand (your right) to grab the butt of the weapon. Turn the barrel towards the assailant while pulling on the butt, and distance yourself from him. (See next technique.)

Throughout the first phase of the technique you must apply pressure and weight to the gun, mainly sideways but also downwards, sending it towards the assailant in order to prevent him from making further use of the weapon.

Threat from the Front – Moving to the "Live" Side

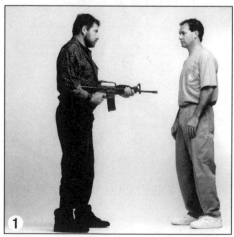

1

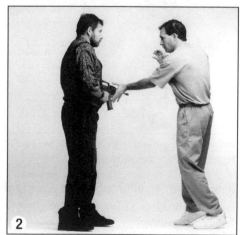

2

The threat is at medium range. The assailant holds the gun in both hands with a strong and steady grip. You choose to apply the technique towards the assailant's "live" side (right side).

Deflect the barrel of the gun, striking it with your open palm. This action "pulls" your body into a forward bend and turn, similar to what occurs when deflecting a stab with a stick or a bayoneted rifle. While deflecting the barrel of the gun, burst diagonally forward.

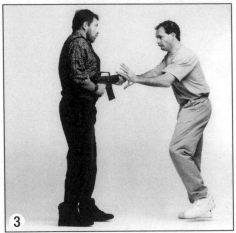

3

While you are bursting forward, as quickly as possible, land the palms of **both** hands, one after the other, on the rifle and grab it.

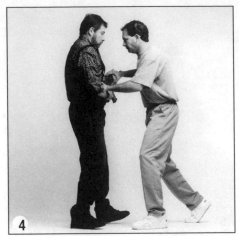

4

Grab the gun and push it diagonally towards the assailant and slightly downward. In doing so, you prevent the assailant from aiming the barrel at you after the initial deflection. You should get **very close** to the gunman's side.

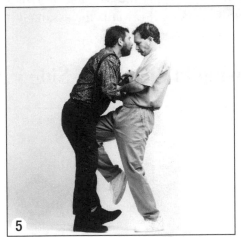

5

Attack the assailant with a knee to his groin; if needed, raise the gun slightly.

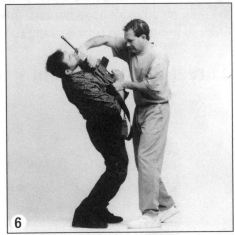

6

Holding the gun firmly, rotate it so that the barrel faces up, directed at the gunman's head.

The technique applied to the assailant's "live" side places you diagonally in front of him, and lets you gain good control of his weapon and assume a good position for counterattack.

The defensive movements here resemble those used for defense against a stab with a stick; they also comprise a deflection of the weapon (position of palm depending on the height of the weapon), body turn, body tilt, and diagonal forward advance.

After deflecting the gun with one hand, your other (rear) hand proceeds to grab the

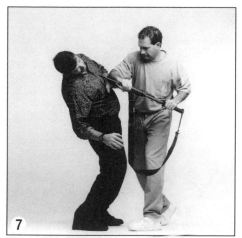

7

Rotate the gun, and at the same time grab it forcefully from the attacker's hands. This action can also serve as an additional counterattack, with the barrel of the gun aimed so as to strike the assailant's head.

gun without giving the assailant time to aim the weapon at you again.

If you need to attack by striking with your hand or elbow, you must do so **only after making sure** that the assailant would find it extremely difficult to move the gun and aim it at you once again.

This is an effective technique against a threat from a distance from the front, or a threat at very close range from the front (although in this case the previous technique may also be highly effective), against a diagonal threat from the side, whether or not at close range, and against a threat to your head or chest.

Threat from the Front – Moving to the "Dead" Side

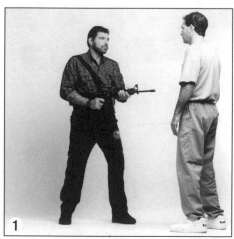

1

The assailant threatens you in a situation where you need to deflect the gun (with your right hand) and move to his "dead" (left) side.

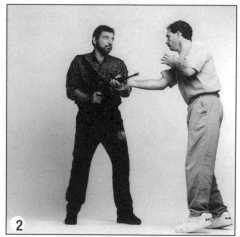

2

Deflect the gun with your right hand, utilizing a body turn, as in *Stab with Stick – Inside Defense from the Outside* (Chap. 3), and burst diagonally forward. Your deflecting hand assists your advance with a slight pull.

When it is necessary to deflect the gun (using your right hand) in the direction that is opposite from the one that is shown in the previous technique, perform a body turn and advance as described above. Then grab the assailant from behind and throw

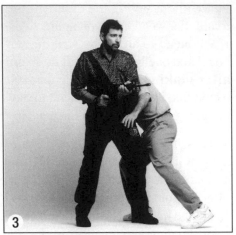

3

Advance to the side and slightly behind the assailant.

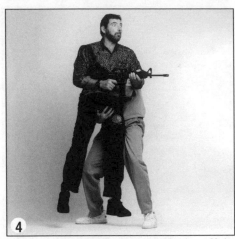

4

Grab the assailant firmly and lift him off the ground, with your body pressed against his, as in the technique for neutralizing a handgun threat in the previous chapter: *Shove and Threat from Behind, at Long Range*.

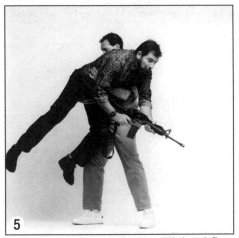

5

Drop the assailant to the ground, head first, pulling with your lower hand and pushing with your upper body.

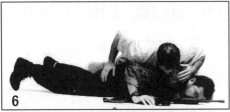

6

Sending both your legs backwards, land on the assailant with a powerful impact.

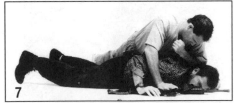

7

As early as possible, counterattack with an elbow strike to the back of the assailant's neck, and grab his weapon.

him, using the same throw that was described in Chapter 4 for neutralizing handgun threat from behind: *Shove and Threat from Behind, at Long Range*.

Hint: It is preferable to deflect the gun while hitting the attacker's wrist or the back of his hand. To lend further assistance while bursting forward, your deflecting hand can add a slight pull at the point of deflection.

Additional Technique: In the situation described here, and **only against a threat with long-barreled rifles and shotguns**, you could perform the basic technique against a handgun threat from the front. (See previous chapter.)

Threat from Behind, at Close Range

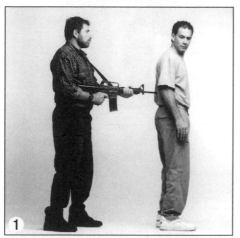

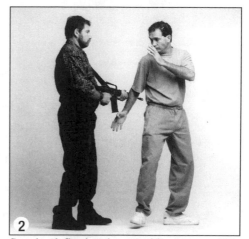

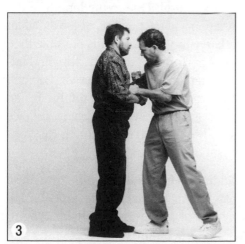

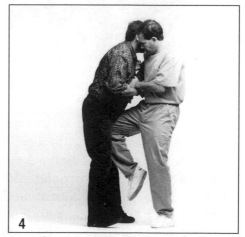

1

The assailant threatens you from behind.

2

Start by deflecting the gun with your arm. This action pulls you into a quick body turn with a burst towards the attacker. Thus, at the start of the deflection, you come close to the attacker.

3

As you burst towards the aggressor (onto the same leg as the defending arm), grab the gun between your forearm, upper arm, hand, and chest (ribs). To enhance control, grab the weapon with your other hand.

4

As early as possible, counterattack with one (or more) knee kicks, usually executed with your front leg after a shuffle with your rear leg.

At the outset, this technique is basically identical to that used in neutralizing a handgun: *Threat from Behind, at Close Range*. When threatened with a long gun

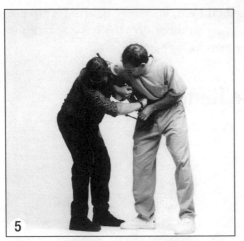

5

With your shoulder and upper body power, start rotating the weapon, sending the barrel towards the assailant's head, in order to hit him.

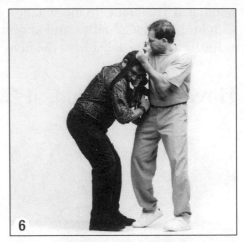

6

If the weapon has a strap attached to it (as it often does), grab the strap and pull it over the assailant's head. Then grab the weapon again with both hands.

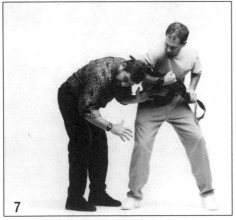

7

Continue with the disarming process.

from behind during the first stage of the technique, you can turn in either direction: to your left or to your right, as required and according to what feels more natural. Due to the length of the weapon and the position of the assailant relative to your body, it is possible that, after performing the body turn and advancing towards the aggressor, you will find yourself at a range suitable for an elbow strike, or even at a longer distance suitable for a straight punch (as your first counterattack).

But, as demonstrated here, if the assailant is holding a **short submachine gun** close to his body, such as around the hip area, you may find that deflecting the gun, turning and advancing may bring you **alongside** the aggressor (rather than **in front** of him) due to the initial shorter distance. In this case, it may be difficult to grab the gun between your arm, forearm, and chest in an effective and safe manner. In such a situation, you can use either of the following variations:

A. This technique depicts a situation where, if your body turn was directed towards the aggressor's "live" side (his right side, in the photograph), you can grab the (deflected) gun in both hands, with one hand (the deflecting hand, as shown here) underneath the gun and the other above it. Then attack by delivering knees to the groin, and disarm the assailant. In this way we have also addressed the problem of an assailant wearing a strap across the body.

Note: If there is any difficulty in removing the shoulder weapon and strap from the assailant, causing a substantial delay, continue to beat the assailant until he is no longer a viable threat. Remember that the gunman may also be **armed with a backup firearm** (such as a concealed handgun). Therefore, act quickly and aggressively in order to terminate the encounter as soon as possible.

B. Turn towards the aggressor's "dead" side (his left side, in the photograph). For more details, see the next technique.

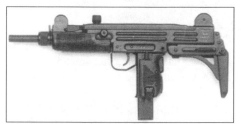

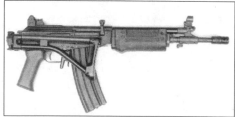

A submachine gun: Uzi SMG.   **A semi-automatic rifle: Galil SAR.**
The photographs of the Uzi SMG and the Galil SAR were printed by courtesy of **Israel Military Industries (I.M.I.)**.

Threat from Behind, at Close Range – Moving to the "Dead" Side

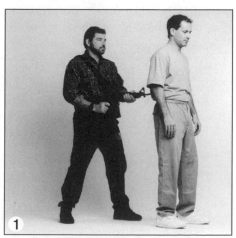

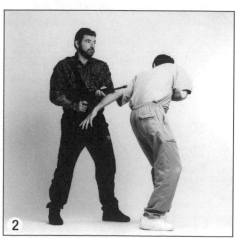

1

The threat, with the gun at your back. According to the situation, you may need (or, for some reason, find it preferable) to turn to your left, towards the assailant's dead side.

2

Deflect the gun, simultaneously turning and advancing towards the gunman. Lower your body while turning, so as not to be pushed by the assailant's (left) forearm or elbow.

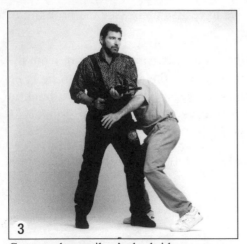

Come to the assailant's dead side.

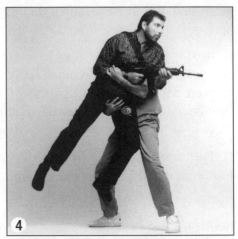

Complete the turn by grabbing and lifting the assailant. (Grabbing the gun instead, is another option you may choose.)

This technique is practically identical to that described (Chap. 4) for neutralizing a handgun threat: *Shove and Threat from Behind, at Long Range*.

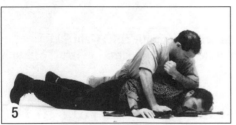

Drop the assailant to the floor, land on him, and counterattack as shown in *Threat from the Front - Moving to the "Dead" Side*.

Against a long gun, you can even utilize the "regular technique", i.e., the basic technique used against a gun threat from the rear. Deflect the gun and grab it with one or two hands and counterattack, first with a punch, an elbow strike, or a knee to the groin.

Hostage Situations

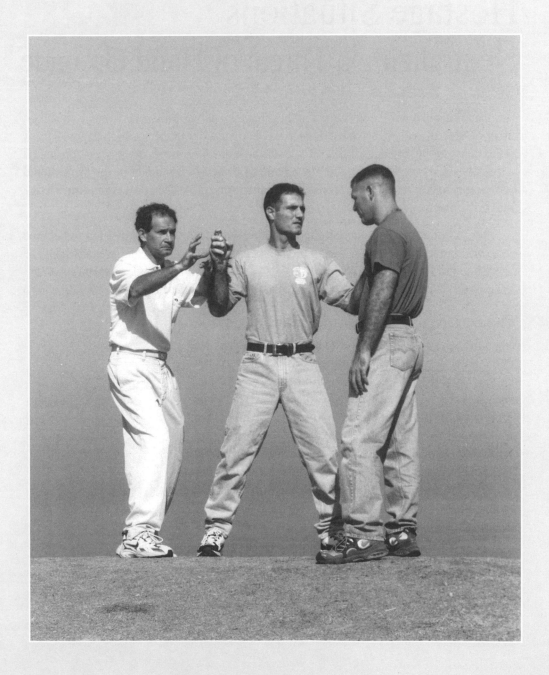

Chapter 6

Hostage Situations
Neutralizing a Threat of Hand Grenade

The situations that will be described in this chapter, such as those encountered in acts of terror or violent crimes, are most dangerous. They usually involve a high degree of risk to the innocent hostages, as well as to the rescue team. Therefore, the material presented in this chapter is intended mainly for **the advanced Krav Maga student or the professional instructor**, and specifically for those **whose duties require the specialized knowledge and skills discussed here**.

In order to understand the tactics and techniques that follow, it is important to become better acquainted with the following physical components of the hand grenade: (1) The safety pin. (2) The lever. (3) The explosive device itself, which includes a spring-operated firing pin, a detonator, explosive material, and the metal (or plastic) casing. (See drawing.)

The Dangerous Aspects of a Hand Grenade

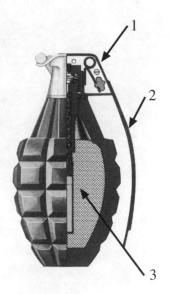

When the safety pin holding the lever is removed, the hand grenade becomes **extremely dangerous**. At the moment the lever is released, it will forcefully leave the grenade. Once the lever is removed, there is nothing to stop the firing pin from striking the detonator. When this happens, the situation is irreversible: **the explosion will occur within two to four seconds**, depending on the type of grenade. If the lever is not removed from the grenade, the detonator will not be activated. The original safety pin (or another, even an improvised one) can be reinserted, and the grenade will not explode.

When a hand grenade explodes in the air, it usually scatters fragments in a spherical manner. When it explodes on the ground, it scatters fragments in a form resembling a hemisphere. The lower fragments will fly low above the ground and rise at a small angle. (See diagram.)

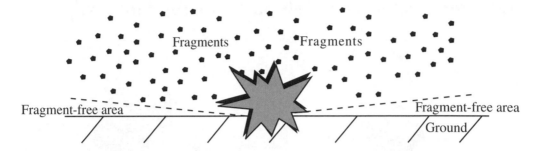

Diagram: Characteristics of explosion when the hand grenade is on the ground.

Possible Situations for Neutralizing Threat of Hand Grenade

A typical threat with a hand grenade might be one where the assailant is holding the grenade in one hand, often with the safety pin removed. How the grenade is brandished depends upon the assailant's wish to impress and instill fear in those around him. Sometimes he will hold the grenade at his side, and in other instances the grenade will be held at or above his shoulder level.

Situations may vary: a threat can be neutralized by one of the persons being threatened, who is part of a group of hostages, or by a member of the rescue team who enters the danger zone for this purpose.

In any incident where a person holding a grenade has taken control, if you decide to take action, **it must be done at maximum speed and with the maximum element of surprise**. One should also bear in mind that in addition to what is anticipated from the assailant or his partners, the hostages may do something or react in some way at the beginning of the rescue action (if they notice it), thus involuntarily revealing the takeover attempt to the "bad guy(s)."

In neutralizing the threat, one who goes to the scene should also take into consideration certain pertinent elements in the immediate vicinity, such as the existence of **mirrors** or the **shadow** he may cast due to the direction of light, which may alert the assailant to his actions or intentions.

According to the above, **the threat must be neutralized as quickly as possible, without "telegraphing" any movement or intention**. One should take action from the moment the decision is made, with determination and without hesitation.

Once you thoroughly understand the following techniques and the principles behind them, practice neutralizing the hand grenade threat when the assailant is in a variety of positions and angles relative to yourself.

Rescuer Comes from Behind – Moving Forward

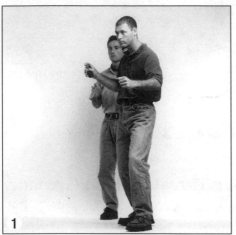

1

The assailant stands with the grenade in his hand, and you come from behind him, moving with momentum. Assume that the safety pin has already been removed from the grenade.

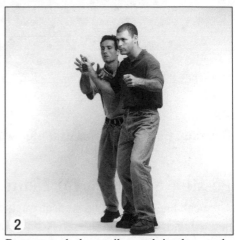

2

Burst towards the assailant and simultaneously, with both your hands, prepare to grab the hand holding the grenade and secure the assailant's wrist and hand. Your forward (left) leg should be the one closer to the opponent.

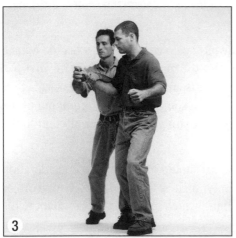

3

By the time that your body reaches the attacker's side, you have grabbed his wrist and hand that is holding the grenade. Be sure to "wrap" the hand holding the grenade, so that the grenade is completely secured, including the operating lever.

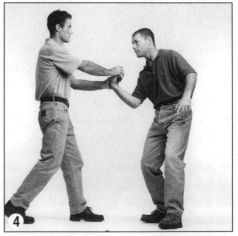

4

In a fast, flowing movement, step forward (on your right leg) and turn towards the opponent. In a continuous movement, switch your legs in preparation for a kick, and begin to apply leverage (called the "cavalier" leverage) to the adversary's wrist.

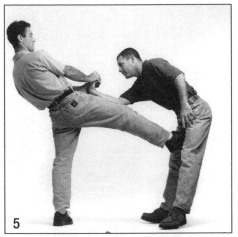

5

Kick the assailant in the groin in order to weaken his resistance.
Note: The kick should be executed in any case, whether or not you encounter resistance.

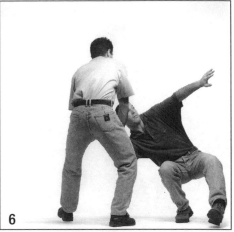

6

Retreat slightly to the rear, and apply a very strong leverage (the same "cavalier" technique) to the attacker's wrist, bending and rotating it outward, pressing down on the hand. This action causes the adversary to lose his balance and immediately fall to the ground.

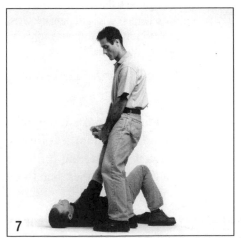

7

The assailant is thrown to the ground, and you stand upright, constantly maintaining control over the hand grenade.

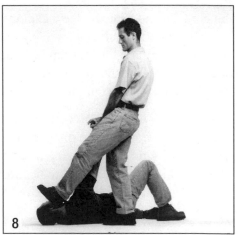

8

Without hesitation, attack again with a kick or stomp to a vulnerable part of the assailant's body. (Aiming at his head is recommended.) Throughout the action, do not loosen your grip on the wrist and hand holding the grenade. Then proceed to remove the grenade from the hand of the now neutralized assailant.

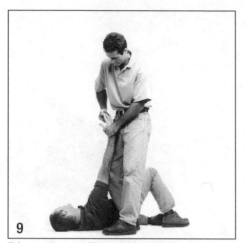

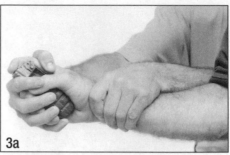

3a

Close-up, photograph 3: Technique for grabbing the hand holding the grenade.

9

Disarm the assailant as detailed further on.

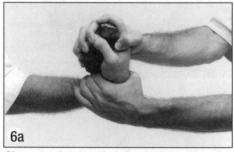

6a

In order to neutralize the threat and the assailant, **you must take the assailant by surprise** by grabbing the hand holding the grenade and applying the technique quickly and efficiently. Optimally, you can approach the assailant from behind,

Close-up, photograph 6: Leverage on the wrist. Holding the assailant's hand, gripping the wrist, bending it, rotating it outward, and applying pressure towards the ground.

or diagonally from behind, or from the side, from the direction of the hand holding the grenade (in the example, from the assailant's right side).

Action from another direction will, of course, be difficult and more dangerous because of the angle, the distance from the grenade, and the assailant's ability to detect your actions. In certain emergency situations (and you should train for those as well), it may be necessary to neutralize the threat from directions other than those recommended, **including from the front**.

Throughout the initial stages of the defense, and until you have disarmed the assailant, it is crucial to maintain a firm grip on the wrist, palm, and fingers of the hand holding the grenade. This is done in order to ensure that the assailant will be prevented from dropping or throwing the grenade! Also, it is extremely important that the lever will not be released during the struggle!

Note: Although the technique demonstrated in the photographs depicts the rescuer kicking the assailant in the groin **before applying the cavalier action**, a well-trained person can apply the cavalier technique sharply and quickly **even without this initial counterattack (kick)**.

This technique should be performed continuously, without any interruptions or pauses. Your initial movement and momentum, together with the cavalier technique, serve to instantly drop the assailant to the ground. The counterattacks used to neutralize the assailant **must be delivered powerfully and with no hesitation**. The assailant should be effectively removed from the equation, and then the hand grenade itself becomes the only immediate concern.

Variation: Neutralization by applying the technique at close range. In this technique, you perform the same stages, but closer to the attacker. Instead of a regular kick, use a knee kick to his groin. This technique will be applied in the event that the assailant is holding the grenade close to his body, if you are in a cramped location and the regular technique cannot be used, or if the assailant pulls his hand back sharply as soon as you grab it.

Taking the Grenade from the Attacker's Hand

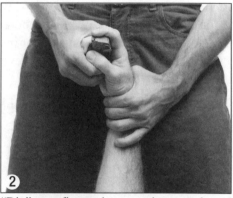

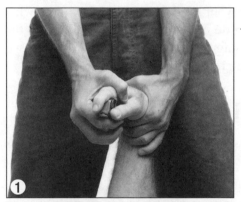

Bend the assailant's hand holding the grenade in order to loosen its grip.

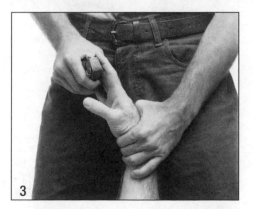

"Dig" your fingers between the grenade and the assailant's palm.

"Dig" into the assailant's palm until you reach the grenade's lever, and grasp it. Throughout this action, **do not let the assailant open his hand. Otherwise, the lever will become separated from the grenade, or the grenade may fall to the ground**. "Peel" the grenade out of the attacker's hand while constantly maintaining pressure on the lever.

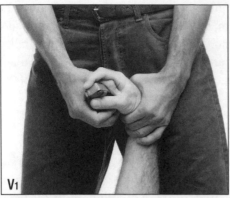

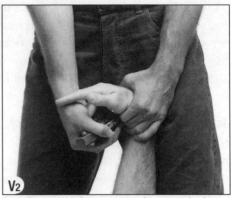

V₁

Alternative technique for taking the grenade out of the attacker's hand: Dig your thumb in deeply between the palm of the assailant's hand and the lever.

V₂

Pressing on the lever, rotate the grenade downwards and remove it from the assailant's hand.

After you have successfully neutralized and disarmed the assailant, you should devote your attention to the "bomb" lying in your hand. You have the two following options: (1) Throw it away, to where it can do no damage. (2) Carefully tape the lever to the body of the grenade, or insert a safety pin (the original or an improvised one) in the appropriate place, to prevent the grenade from exploding.

Rescuer Comes from Behind – Pulling Backwards

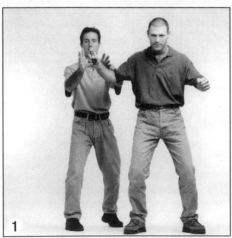

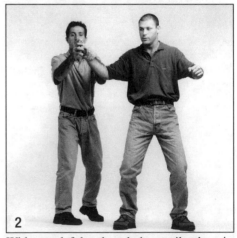

1

Similar to the previous technique, you lunge from behind the attacker, intending to grab his wrist and the palm of his hand holding the grenade. In order to make the pull backwards more effective, your right foot must be in front.

2

With your left hand, grab the assailant's wrist forcefully, and at the same time "wrap" the palm of your right hand around the palm of the attacker's and the grenade. **As early as possible**, start pulling to the rear.

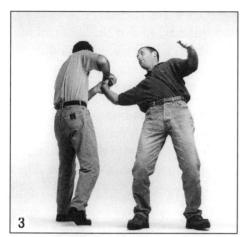

Forcefully pull the palm of the assailant's hand (and the grenade) to the rear, while applying downward pressure, i.e., creating a leverage action on the assailant's wrist. In doing so, you turn to the rear and even retreat, with your rear leg (the left leg in this case) in order to increase the force of the action.

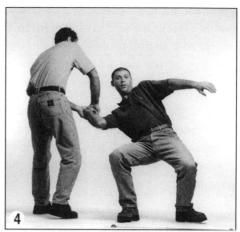

Create a strong leverage on the assailant's wrist. From the force of the pull and the leverage, the attacker falls backwards; the grenade passes in close proximity beside his shoulder.

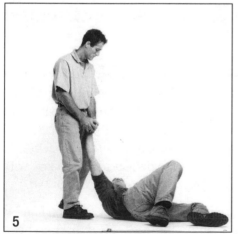

The assailant reaches the ground. Be aware that up to this moment, he has not actually been attacked.

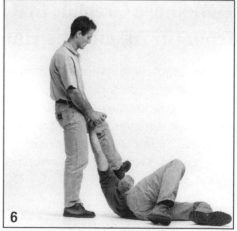

Attack him instantly with a kick, for example, a stomping kick to the assailant's head, and proceed to disarm him as described earlier.

This technique is usually executed in a place and situation in which you cannot, in one or two steps, get in front of the assailant, such that you cannot execute the previous technique, e.g., in a crowded bus or an airplane aisle, near a wall, or in other confined spaces.

You should grab the palm of the assailant's hand, so as to make it possible to create the leverage on his wrist. Practice this grab under varying conditions, for instance, when the grenade is held high or low. The pull backwards causes the assailant to lose his balance. You must **perform this action quickly**, so that the assailant will not be able to turn towards you or straighten his elbow, which would neutralize the leverage action and keep him from falling backwards. Execute the pull in such a way that the grenade passes close to the side of the assailant's shoulder.

If the assailant falls and pulls his hand forcefully towards his body, you will need to execute knee kicks to his head or ribs, or strike his face with the secured grenade in order to overcome his pull and be able to stand erect. Once you are in a standing position above the assailant, you can kick him or stomp him in the head. Then disarm him.

Note: This type of leverage action on the assailant's wrist, intended to take him backwards, can also be used when you try to perform the first technique in this chapter. When you are trying to apply this technique, and the attacker, feeling the grasp, strongly pulls back his hand (with your hands) towards himself, **you must move with his pull** and simultaneously apply the leverage action to the rear, towards the assailant's back and downward. Your hands will pass by the side of his shoulders, sending him flat on his back.

Handling a Grenade that has been Activated or Dropped from the Assailant's Hand

During the neutralization stage, once the lever has been released, the grenade is activated and the process becomes irreversible. In such a case, you must **grab the grenade quickly and roll it, throw it, or put it anywhere that the explosion will not cause damage**. Then move away quickly by running or rolling for cover. If possible, lie flat on your stomach, with your legs crossed, heels in the direction of the grenade. **You should also warn others** nearby of the danger of explosion, with a loud cry such as "EVERYBODY DOWN!", "HAND GRENADE!", or "BOMB!"

Note: At times, it might be advisable to secure the grenade that has dropped and is about to explode, underneath the assailant's body, but **only after he has been completely neutralized** by your counterattack, i.e., cannot move and is no longer a real threat.

Neutralizing a Threat of Handgun

Threat from the Front

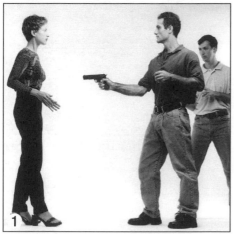

A hostage's life is being threatened. Your position relative to the assailant's allows you to burst towards the gunman, diagonally from the rear.

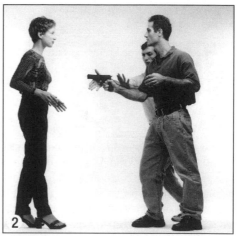

Burst forward, sending both hands towards the gun and the assailant's hand holding it. Your body stays behind.

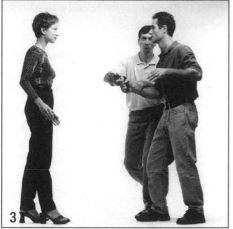

Deflect and redirect the gun's line of fire, and grab it with your front (right) hand. At the same time, with your rear (left) hand, grasp and slightly pull the forearm (near the wrist) of the hand holding the gun. Using both hands, start applying a powerful leverage action on the gun and onto the assailant's hand holding it.

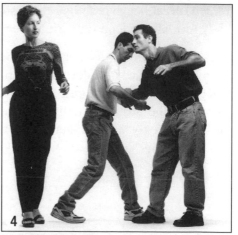

Instantly rotate the gun towards the assailant, using the turning momentum and the power of your entire body. This you do, while stepping with your rear (right) leg and turning towards the attacker. The barrel of the gun is sent under the assailant's forearm in order to allow for an efficient disarming.

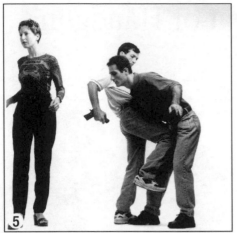

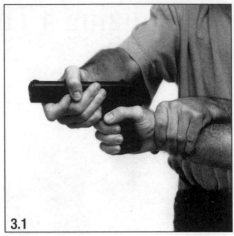

Finish disarming the gunman, and counterattack simultaneously by kicking or kneeing him in the groin. You can continue to counterattack while retreating, after the disarming stage. As the actions of the hostage cannot be foreseen, do not rely on him (or her) to make any particular move. In this case, the hostage starts to retreat.

Close-up, photograph 3: Deflecting and grabbing the gun.

The action of grabbing and deflecting the gun in this technique also resembles the technique used in neutralizing a handgun threat: ***Threat from the Side, in Front of Your Arm***, although grabbing the assailant's wrist is executed differently here. The body turn allows for a powerful leverage on the assailant's hand and wrist.

The approach to the assailant and the capturing of his weapon are similar to the actions performed in order to neutralize a threat from a hand grenade. Note that in this case, **grabbing the gun follows the deflection of the line of fire** (the barrel). Here too, the hostage's behavior cannot be predicted, and therefore the rescuer must act quickly and then get the hostage to a safe place, according to the situation and the rescuer's own position.

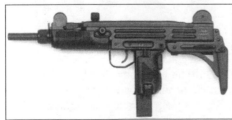

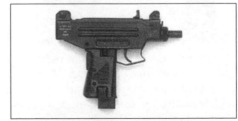

A submachine gun: Mini Uzi SMG.   **A semi-automatic gun: Uzi Pistol**.
The photographs of the Mini Uzi and the Uzi Pistol were printed by courtesy of **Israel Military Industries (I.M.I.)**.

Threat to the Head – Assailant is Holding the Hostage

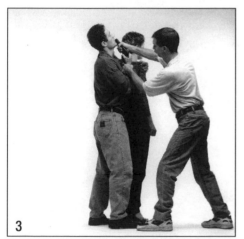

The gunman is holding the hostage, threatening with his handgun to the victim's head. You, the rescuer, approach the assailant diagonally from the rear.

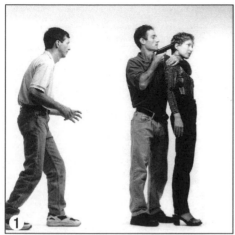

Deflect and grab the gun, with one hand (your right) as your rear (left) hand pulls and grabs the gunman's wrist. As in the previous technique, step to the side or in front of the assailant.

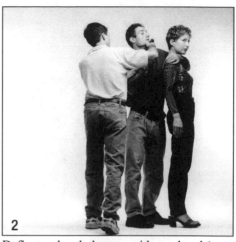

Continue your step as you send the gun towards the assailant's face. Striking him with the barrel of the gun is a by-product of this action and should not have any major effect on the time it takes to disarm him.

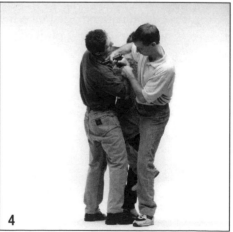

Counterattack with your rear (right) knee as you continue rotating the handgun in the assailant's hand, sending it backwards and down.

Note: Photographs 3-5 were taken from diagonally behind the assailant.

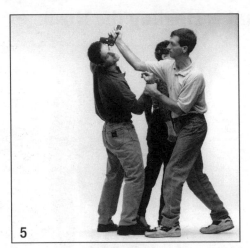

5

Continue counterattacking, possibly striking
the assailant with the gun.

This technique is basically identical to the previous one, though in this case, the
shorter distance between the assailant and the hostage makes it more difficult for
the rescuer to deflect the gun and disarm the assailant.

After the counterattacks, distance the hostage from the assailant and, if possible,
leave the scene together with the hostage to a safer location (if he or she has not
already moved away).

Using Everyday Objects as Defensive Weapons

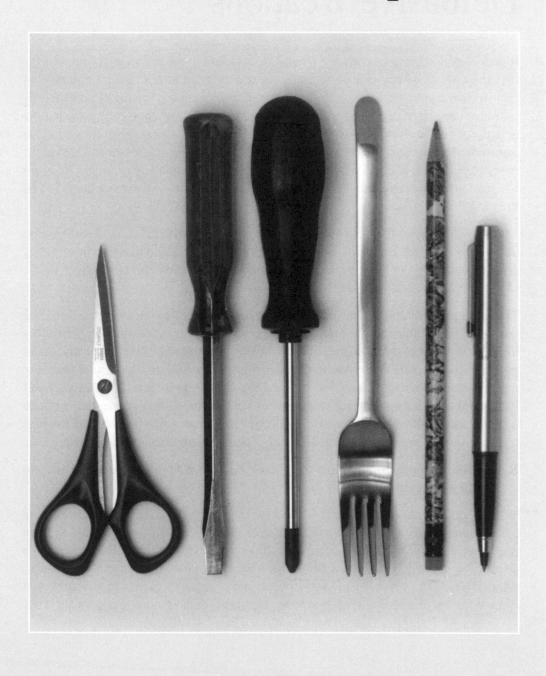

Chapter 7

Using Everyday Objects as Defensive Weapons

In self-defense, great importance should be attached to the use of everyday objects that may be found on your person or near the scene of attack. Select objects that can improve your performance in either defense or attack (or both) and thereby increase the effectiveness of your actions. Using such a weapon in response to an aggressor can provide you with additional options for action. With the aid of an improvised weapon, it is easier to foil dangerous acts by the aggressor and overcome more than one assailant. Besides, by brandishing the weapon aggressively in order to make an impressive show of strength, the confrontation sometimes can even be prevented altogether!

You should think of the weapon available to you as an **integral part of your body**, and not as external, limiting accessory. You must be quick and decisive in selecting a suitable object, and your choice should enable you to make the most effective use of this object against the specific danger you are facing.

The greater the surprise achieved by the assailant, the lesser your chances of finding and using a suitable object. The more expected the attack, and the longer it takes the assailant to reach you, the better the opportunity to locate and retrieve an improvised weapon. Therefore, if you fear a surprise attack in a particular location, e.g., between your apartment and the parking garage, **you should equip yourself in advance with appropriate items** such as a canister of tear gas, a heavy bunch of keys, etc. Although these items should be easily accessible, sometimes the best move will be to **run a few yards to where there is something you can use**.

Remember: You should familiarize yourself with objects that are available to you along often-traveled routes.

When a confrontation is expected, and especially if the attacker (or attackers) are very powerful, it is recommended that you equip yourself **in advance** with an improvised weapon that will afford you the greatest measure of defense (such as a stick or a stone). You should **hold the object in your hand**, ready to use it. Otherwise, if the object is in your pocket, purse, or briefcase, for example, you have little chance of reaching it in time, particularly if you are taken by surprise.

Note: As a strict rule, use your weapon in such a way that there is little chance that it will fall into the hands of the opponent, who might then use it against you!

Caution: In some countries it may be **illegal to arm yourself in advance with certain weapons** as described above.

Note: Utilizing a weapon-like object for defensive purposes is definitely appropriate in situations where your life and physical well-being are in actual danger. On the other hand, escalating unnecessarily to a higher force option may eventually result in civil or criminal liability!

Incidentally, even when the potential assailant is an animal, such as a large dog, your chances will be better if you are equipped with a rock or stick as a weapon, or a chair or other large object that can serve as a shield.

Everyday objects are used according to their shape and characteristics. For our purposes, we divide them into the following categories:

Stick-like objects

Using these items, you can attack with swings or stabs. (See beginning of Chap. 3: **Defense against an Assailant Armed with a Stick**.) Aim at a vulnerable point on the attacker's body, and attack, as necessary in accordance with the circumstances. If you are using a heavy stick, it is preferable to attack with strikes and swings, but if you have a thin, light or flimsy stick that is easily broken, stabs are more effective.

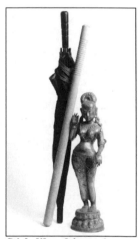

If you hold the stick so that a small part of it (about 1 to 2 inches) protrudes behind your hand, this part can be used for attack at close range, e.g., *hammer punches*. The stick is also an excellent means to defend yourself against the aggressor's attacks. (This will be discussed later in the section on shield-like objects.)

Stick-like objects: baton, umbrella, heavy statue.

Stick-like objects: An umbrella, a tall vase, a fireplace poker, a PR-24 (police baton with perpendicular handle), and other club-like objects such as a baseball bat, a rolling pin, a tree branch, a mop or broom handle, a pipe wrench, etc.

Stone-like objects

A stone can be thrown from a distance, and can also be held in your hand and used as a weapon for delivering punches. **Any heavy, relatively small object held in your hand can help by increasing the force of the strike and adding to its range and impact**.

The method for attacking with a stone that is held in your hand is usually the **overhead hammer punch**. However, you can also use the stone for actions resembling a **straight punch**, a **roundhouse "hook" punch**, or a **lateral strike**. When throwing the stone at a target, we will utilize its momentum from back to front, similar to the way one throws a baseball. Complete the throw by executing a pointing move and turning your shoulder towards the target.

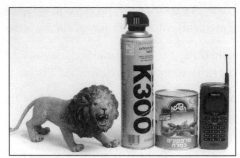

Stone-like objects: heavy plastic toy, insect spray (can be used either as an impact weapon or as toxic material for injuring the assailant's face and eyes), can, cellular phone.

Remember: If your attack or throw proves ineffective, the adversary may make use of the stone against you! Obviously, the idea is **not** to allow the stone or any other object to be used against you. Therefore, your throw must be executed at a distance, range, height, and speed that will prove effective.

A variety of **stone-like objects**, such as an ashtray, a heavy tumbler, a statuette, a bottle (especially a glass bottle filled with liquid), a plate (which can be thrown like a Frisbee), etc., may be easily found nearby, in various locations.

Small objects

Small, relatively light objects can be used to distract the aggressor's attention, usually without causing him any serious harm. Throwing a handful of coins, your wrist watch, a small bunch of keys, etc., at the assailant's face will surprise him, hamper his activity, and perhaps hit him in the eyes. Distracted, he will be momentarily vulnerable to your attack.

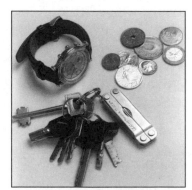

Small objects: wrist watch, handful of coins, bunch of keys.

A Real-Life Story

Ruth, a young Israeli soldier, had taken a brief course in Krav Maga. One evening, while on her way home from the army base, a man sprang at her from the bushes beside the road, grabbed her by the arms and clothing and began pulling her into the bushes. Once the young woman recovered from the momentary shock, she moved towards the assailant and kicked him in the groin. When he bent over from the pain, she picked up a rock, struck him on the head with it, and fled.

Throwing a Small Object against an Attack or Threat with a Knife

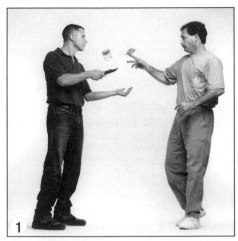

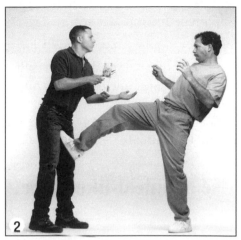

The assailant prepares to stab or is standing in front of you, holding a knife in a threatening manner. Throw something at him, at eye level, while advancing towards him as needed.

The surprised assailant will react to the object hurtling towards his eyes. This natural reaction, closing his eyes or shifting his weight backwards, will expose the assailant to a kick in the groin.

This technique is very important in a threatening or fighting atmosphere, against slashing and any other form of stabbing, when the assailant is still at the preliminary stages of his attack. You can distract the aggressor's attention and focus by throwing any small object at his face, especially at his eyes. The object may be a set of keys, a bunch of papers, a handkerchief, a handful of coins, a wrist watch, etc. Simultaneously with the throw, advance and attack with a regular kick to the assailant's groin at maximum range and with great force, tilting your upper body back. Follow with additional attacks, according to the angle and circumstances. (See Chap. 1: **Defense against Knife Attack**.)

Remember: It is usually ineffective to throw an object at an assailant engaged in the midst of a powerful attack, unless the item is **heavy enough** to stop him or hinder his progress.

Shield-like objects

The purpose of the shield is to stop or deflect the attack. The shield can be **rigid**, such as a stick, a wooden board, a chair, or the metal lid of a trash can or a large saucepan. It can also be **soft**, such as a shoulder bag, a briefcase, a large parcel, etc.

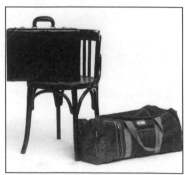

Shield-like objects: travel bag, briefcase, chair.

With a shield-like object it is even possible to hinder the assailant's progress or "stop him in his tracks." For example, a large object thrown at the attacker's feet can serve as an obstacle; locking a door or slamming it in his face can stop him altogether and may also cause him some harm; or a car door thrust opened forcefully at the opportune moment can trip an aggressor or stop him cold.

This principle can also be applied to defending against **two assailants**. In this case, your objective is to position yourself at an angle, relative to that of your opponents, which will cause one of them to hinder the actions of the other. Sometimes you can push one of them against the other, using the first attacker's body as a shield or as a means to hamper the progress of the other. (See Chap. 10: **Defense against Two Armed Assailants**.)

Use of shield-like object: chair

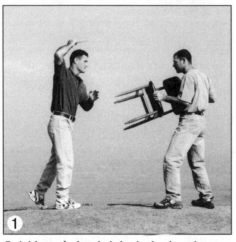

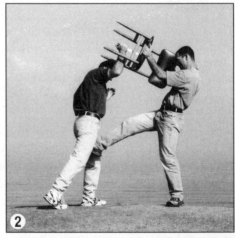

Quickly grab the chair by its back and seat.

Using the chair as a shield and thrusting it in the direction of the attack. From beneath the chair, counterattack with a regular kick to the assailant's groin.

The situation shown above (in photograph 1) should be achieved using a rapid, economical movement. According to the distance and timing, grasp the chair and lift it, for instance, while retreating to a distance that permits more effective action.

The most convenient and natural hold on the chair will usually be the one shown in the photograph. Under other conditions, e.g., to maintain a greater distance, you can hold only the back of the chair. If the chair is backless, hold it by its seat. Sometimes it may be preferable to grip the chair by its legs or in any other suitable manner that fits your position.

The chair (or any other shield-like object) is directed against the attack with the intent to stop or deflect it. The chair affords the defender with a tremendous reach advantage. It can help stop a knife or stick attack, defend against a kick, etc.

The counterattack must fit the relative angle and the specific situation. It can be executed with the chair itself, by kicking below the chair, or even, if needed, by a punch (after releasing your grip on the chair).

The chair can also be used for **attacking**. It can be used to deliver strikes, like a stick. It can be waved as a threat or held in front of the assailant (even a vicious dog) and it can be thrust in a straight stabbing movement, with its legs aimed at the adversary's body.

Various objects can also be used to delay the aggressor for a moment, giving you time to flee the scene and avoid an undesired encounter. For example, overturning a table onto an assailant who is approaching you, or throwing it into his path.

Knife-like objects

A knife, or a similar object, can be used for **both** defensive actions and counterattacks, by stabbing or slashing actions. The basic method for using the knife is described in chapter 1.

Knife-like objects: A broken bottle, a pencil, a pen, a screwdriver, a pair of scissors, a sharp piece of metal, a short club, a knitting needle, etc. Duller, less durable objects should be used only for stabbing at a suitable vulnerable point on the adversary's body.

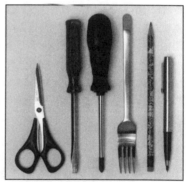

Knife-like objects: scissors, screwdrivers, fork, pencil, pen.

Rope-like objects

Such weapons (belt, rope, whip, rolled-up towel, etc.), can be used to lash, entwine, strike, or tie up the attacker. Possible types of attack are brandishing the object, rotating it, delivering lashing blows with it. Rope-like objects can also be used to tie up the assailant after neutralizing him. Some armies still teach how to tie up an enemy soldier with improvised means such as a rope, a shoelace, or a belt.

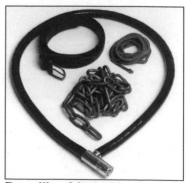

Rope-like objects: bicycle chain with a lock, belt, chain, rope.

Liquids and sprays

Some **liquids**, especially caustic or toxic chemicals, can be used effectively against an attacker, in addition to the element of surprise that is inherent in them. Slinging a common alcoholic beverage, a cup of hot coffee or a bowl of boiling soup into the aggressor's face can have an immediate effect, making him vulnerable to further attack.

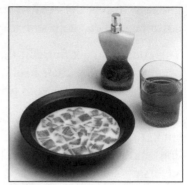

Various **sprays**, directed at the assailant's face, can make him close his eyes and might cause him serious damage, depending on the substance used. Even a handful of sand, which is thrown in the aggressor's eyes, can stun him

Strong liquids: liquors, chemicals, hot liquids.

and momentarily impede his progress, leaving him vulnerable to attack.

Objects of combined characteristics used as improvised weapons

As noted earlier, various objects can be used as improvised weapons in different situations: for attack only, for defense only, in a combination of both defense and attack, or as a means of distracting the assailant's attention, thereby allowing you to counterattack or escape. With the following objects, note also how different characteristics and categories are sometimes combined in a single weapon.

Bayoneted rifle: A combination of the categories of an edged weapon (knife) and a stick. An ax and a spear represent a similar combination.

Throwing a sharp piece of glass or a knife: This is a combination of a stone and a knife.

Chair: Presents a combination of shield and stick, which can also be used to attack in various ways, as explained previously in this chapter.

Throwing a spear, sharp stick, or pitchfork: This is a combination of stone, knife, and stick.

Other categories of weapons include, but are not limited to, flaming or heated objects, elements carrying high voltage, and even a motor vehicle (which can be used as a lethal weapon to deliver serious bodily harm or even death).

Intimidating your opponent

One of the greatest advantages of using an improvised weapon for self-defense, is that such an object can be used to aggressively threaten or exhibit so much strength and danger to the assailant, that **he will be intimidated and change his mind**

about attacking. For example, if you are holding a walking stick and wave it powerfully at the assailant, chances are good that he will retreat and avoid confrontation.

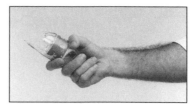

Intimidation: holding a broken bottle

Summary

As a student of Krav Maga, you must become accustomed to quickly scanning your immediate environment for objects that can be used as improvised weapons should the need arise. When you come to a new place, survey the area thoroughly, noting any objects nearby that could prove useful.

Similar to an expert chef who is capable of preparing a gourmet meal from various ingredients that he finds in his refrigerator, you should be ready to "cook" for an occasional assailant from an impressive and effective "menu" of your own, using standard, everyday objects that you can find within reach.

Practice the correct use of various objects. This should include the following skills: accuracy in throwing both light and heavy objects at a small target, executing strikes or stabs with a stick, defending with shield-like objects, etc.

A Real-Life Story

Diane, a woman in her fifties, attended a workshop intended to increase public awareness of self-defense. After the lecture, she asked the instructor the following question: "I am not trained in Krav Maga, and I am really frightened, especially when leaving the office late at night and walking to my car in the parking garage. What should I do if I am attacked on the way to or from the office or my car?" As tear gas and O.C. spray were virtually impossible to obtain at the time, the instructor advised her to carry a small portable fire extinguisher (of the type that fits into the glove compartment of a car), and hold it in her hand from the moment she leaves the office until she is inside her car (or vice versa). "The fire extinguisher must be ready for action, and not just sitting in your purse," the instructor stressed. Diane took his advice, and a few weeks later it really proved effective: She succeeded in foiling such an attack by spraying the contents of the fire extinguisher into the assailant's face.

Short Stick against
Knife Attack

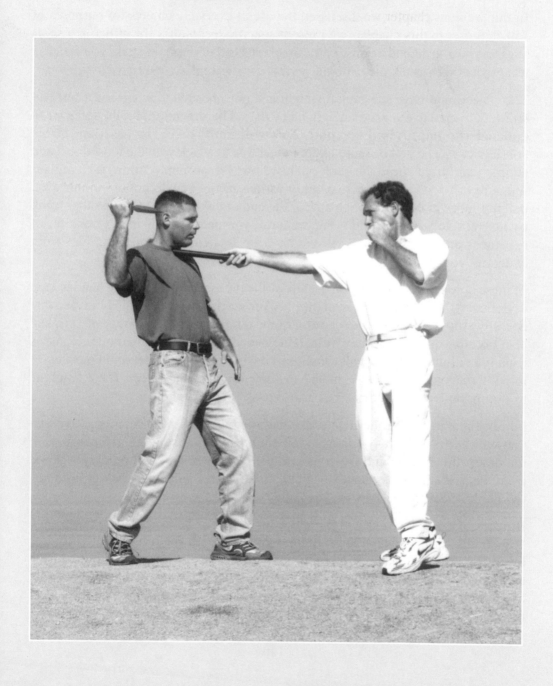

Chapter 8

Short Stick against Knife Attack

In the previous chapter we discussed the use of everyday objects for purposes of self-defense. In this chapter, we present specific techniques for utilizing a short stick in order to defend against knife attack. Instead of the short stick, you can also use objects such as a knife, a bottle, a vase, or any similarly improvised weapon.

The object must have substantial weight and must be able to withstand a forceful strike delivered to the assailant's hand (wrist). **The defender should attempt to conceal the improvised weapon**. This will not deprive the assailant of his confidence and he will be more likely to feel free to attack with the most direct and simple stab. If you hold the stick openly, however, you may "draw the assailant into a fight", and he is likely to employ various tactics and deceptions to make the defense more problematic. (See note at the end of this chapter.) On the other hand, by aggressively brandishing your weapon, you put yourself into a position of readiness and this may also intimidate your assailant, discouraging him from attacking you altogether.

In these defense techniques, you usually strike the assailant's stabbing hand to stop or deflect it. You aim this strike at the attacker's wrist area, since this is an area that is easily stopped or deflected (because of the distance and the leverage effect), and also because this area is more vulnerable, since it has little fat and muscle and is usually unclothed. The overall technique consists of a body defense, in most cases moving diagonally sideways, and a hand defense using the object. These combine to stop or deflect the attack at the earliest possible moment.

It is essential to execute the counterattack **immediately** after the defense! Therefore, you will perform the two actions at maximum speed, integrating one action with the other: the defense and the counterattack. In effect, you will quickly proceed from the strike to the assailant's hand to strike another vulnerable part of his body, usually his neck or his head.

If necessary, and especially if the attack takes you by surprise and comes from a "problematic" direction, you can **defend yourself with the forearm of your free hand**, i.e., the one that is not holding the improvised weapon, using one of the techniques demonstrated in the first chapter: **Defense against Knife Attack**. Simultaneously with or immediately after the defense, execute a counterattack, using the short stick or another "regular" attack technique, e.g., a kick, punch, etc.

Defense against Oriental Stab

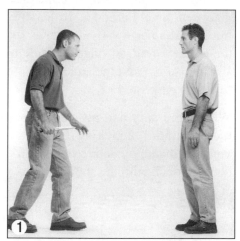

1

Start from a neutral stance. If possible, conceal the improvised weapon from the assailant.

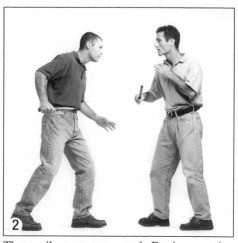

2

The assailant moves to attack. Begin executing a downward strike with your stick, aiming at your adversary's wrist area. At the same time, apply a body defense by turning and advancing diagonally to the side.

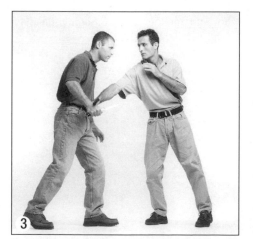

3

Stop the attacker's hand at the wrist. A split second before hitting the attacker's hand, you must grip your stick firmly, preparing for the downward strike.

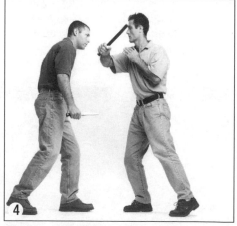

4

Continue immediately with another strike, to the assailant's head.

At the same time that you evade the attack, you stop it at a safe distance from your body, using the stick. You will use the same technique against attack with a knife held in the assailant's left hand. The stopping action is executed with a direct downward motion, grasping the stick tightly in your hand. For this action to succeed, the short stick must be sufficiently heavy and sturdy.

The counterattack with the stick can be a horizontal swing to the side, hitting the assailant's head, like a slashing attack, or a stabbing movement aimed at the base of the assailant's throat, right in the hollow between the collarbones. If the stick impacts at a narrow spot, such as the top of the throat, its edge is liable to slip, and as a result the attack will not fulfill its purpose.

When necessary and possible, block the assailant's attacking hand with your free hand, by delivering the first counterattack with the short stick.

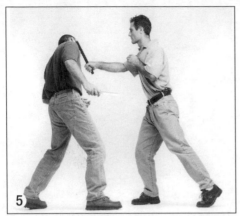

Hit the temple area of your opponent with a slashing type of attack or use a stabbing strike at the base of his throat, or to another highly vulnerable area that is open to attack. You might perform an additional counterattack, e.g., a regular kick to the assailant's groin with your left leg, or a straight left punch, **all according to the angle and range between you and the assailant**; then move away quickly.

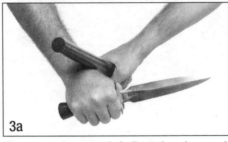

Close-up, photograph 3: Stopping the attack at the assailant's wrist.

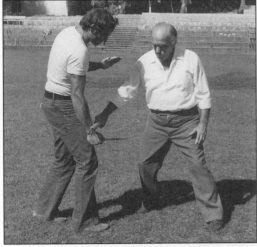

Grandmaster Imi demonstrating a defense against an upward stab, using a short and heavy stick to stop the attacking forearm.

Defense against Regular Stab

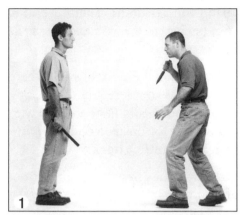

1

Starting from a neutral, passive position. As demonstrated here, the stick is neither hidden nor shown in a threatening manner. (See note at the end of this chapter.)

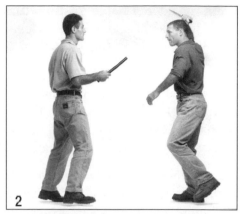

2

The assailant attacks. Begin immediately with a stabbing counterattack, utilizing the reach of the stick. Move diagonally forward and sideways to put yourself outside the line of attack.

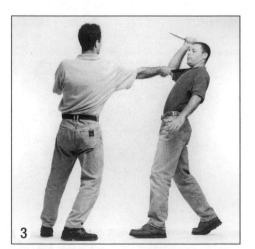

3

You stop the attacker at a distance by sending a straight "stab" to the base of his throat, while executing a body turn and advancing diagonally sideways with a short step. Your next move can be, for example, to attack him with a regular kick to the groin.

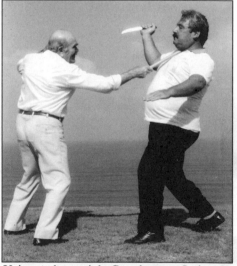

Using a short stick, Grandmaster Imi stops an assailant bursting forward and trying to attack him with a downward stab.

In this technique **timing** is a very important factor; correct timing is necessary in order to stop the assailant at a safe distance. "Stabbing" with the stick stops the attacker abruptly. The turning of your body, as well as the advancing movement diagonally forward, establishe a better range for action and a good body defense.

Note: As shown here, it is possible to aim your attack at the clavicle hollow between the collarbones, as this is the wider part of the neck; if the stick impacts at a narrow point, its edge is liable to **slip without injuring the assailant**. Therefore, it is sometimes preferable to immediately use a strike (swing) to the assailant's head as the initial counterattack, hitting him diagonally downwards.

If the attack has taken you by surprise or came at you from your right side (where your weapon is located), you can use the stick or either of your forearms (depending on the angle) to defend against the attacking hand. You should then proceed with counterattacks, consistent with the principle illustrated for the technique *Defense against Oriental Stab*. (See Chap. 1: **Defense against Knife Attack**.)

Depending on the nature of the attack and whether it comes from the front or from your left side (your unarmed hand), another option may be to defend with the technique that utilizes the forearm of your free hand, and, as early as possible, to launch a counterattack, using the stick as an impact weapon. (See the last section of this chapter.)

Defense against Straight Stab

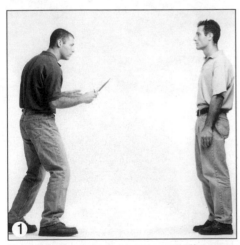

Start from a neutral stance, concealing your improvised weapon from the opponent's view.

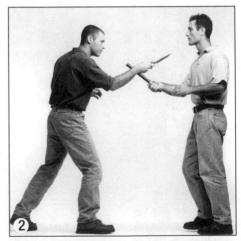

With a fast, strong strike, deflect the stabbing hand in the vicinity of the wrist. The deflecting hand leads your body defense, "pulling" your body into a turn and a small step diagonally to the side, thus evading the line of attack.

Note: It is extremely important **to use proper timing when deflecting the attacker's stabbing hand**. The reasons for striking at the assailant's wrist are specified at the beginning of this chapter.

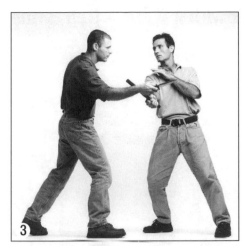

The complete defensive action.

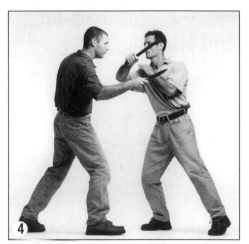

Immediately proceed with a fast counterattack, for example, a horizontal strike.

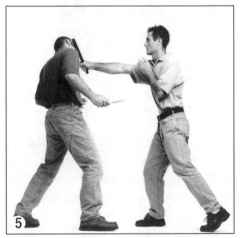

Hit the assailant's head, in the temple area, and then counterattack again or move out of the danger zone.

Another technique: If you have been attacked from the side or diagonally from the side (where your improvised weapon is located), you will use an outside defense technique, e.g., holding the stick in your right hand. When the assailant stabs at you from this angle, you should execute an outside defense, simultaneously advancing diagonally forward on your left leg. This is done in order to remove your body from the line of attack and create a safe distance from which to operate. (See a similar technique: *Straight Stab – Deflecting by Outside Defense*, in the next chapter: **Stick against Stick**.)

Defense against Slashing Attack with a Knife – Retreating and Kicking

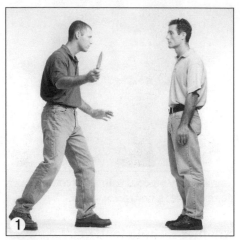

The assailant executes a slashing attack, aimed at your throat.

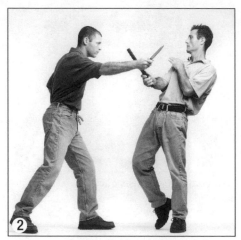

Lean your torso backwards. If necessary, you can retreat, stepping slightly to the rear, on one foot (the one opposite the hand holding the stick, in this case, the left foot), while stopping the assailant's hand by striking with your stick. You are now ready to kick.

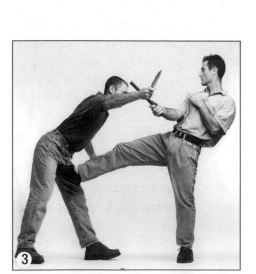

As your first counterattack, deliver a kick to the assailant's groin, and continue as needed with an additional kick or by using the stick.

This simple technique is based on the natural reaction of retreating in order to put yourself outside the danger zone. To this reaction, we add the action of stopping the attack through use of the stick. Your initial reaction of retreating to the rear should serve as a complete defense; that is, the knife will pass you by and will not harm you, even without the stick defense. This retreat may include a small step backwards along with a backward lean of your torso, while the kick is sent as quickly and as early as possible to a vulnerable point on the assailant's body.

Defense against Slashing Attack – Acting after the Knife has Passed You

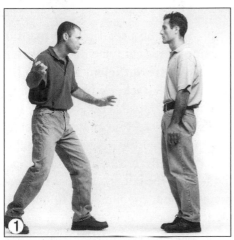

The assailant executes a slashing attack, for example, towards your throat or face. You begin from a passive stance and, if possible, conceal your weapon.

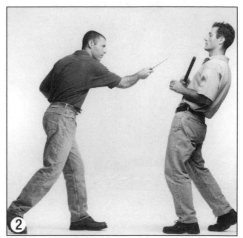

Retreat with a step backwards and lean with your upper body backwards in order to put yourself beyond the range of the knife, at the same time raising your hands defensively on guard. The knife has passed, and your back heel is raised.

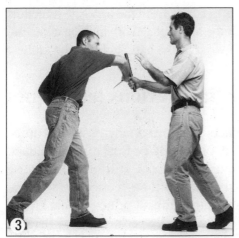

The assailant returns with another slashing attack, but this time you are more prepared. Using the stick (and if necessary your other hand too), stop the attacking hand, which is now moving from the assailant's left side to his right. This defensive action precedes the return of your body (from the leaning-back position), as well as a step forward.

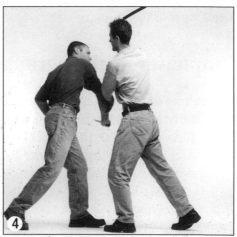

As fast as possible, advance and grab the assailant's forearm with your free hand, and begin counterattacking.

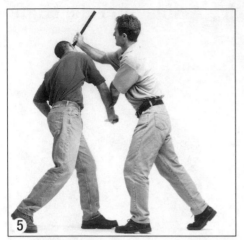

5

Execute a forceful attack to a vulnerable point on the assailant's body while preventing him from making any further use of the knife.

This technique uses first the natural reaction of retreat, when the defender **does not have sufficient time** to fully react to the attacker's first slash, and leaning backwards, he is raising his hands defensively on guard (but not in an action geared towards stopping the attack). While retreating backwards, the heel of the defender's rear foot remains raised, enabling him to quickly switch to the counterattack.

If the backward retreat was large-scale, more and more weight will be transferred to the rear, and the previous technique (*Defense against Slashing Attack with a Knife – Retreating and Kicking*) will be appropriate, though this time it will be directed against the **second** slashing movement.

After the knife has passed, and while it returns to attack from the opposite direction, you are ready to stop the attack, whether with the aid of the short stick or with your hand, sent to the assailant's forearm or to the wrist of the hand holding the knife.

Emphases in photographs for the previous techniques

In teaching these techniques to soldiers or others who are serving in **special units**, we usually emphasize the techniques that may ultimately be fatal to the assailant. Therefore, practicing those techniques in this framework will include the use of a knife, as well as a short stick. The knife is a deadly though effective weapon, and therefore is essential for those operating on the biblical principle that killing in self-defense while in life-or-death situations is morally permissible. (Literally: *If anyone comes to kill you, you should kill him first.*)

If you are using a knife against an oriental (upward) stab or a straight stab, your counterattack can take one of the following two forms: either stabbing or slashing at the assailant's face or throat.

Remember: After your counterattack, it may still be possible for the assailant to strike again. Be sure to continue in a manner that will enable you to maintain a good defensive position.

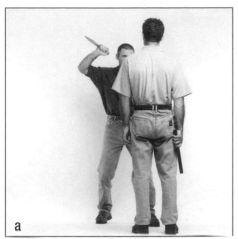

a

Initial stance; this photograph was taken from behind the defender. It is advised to keep the weapon well hidden from the attacker's view, giving him no reason to employ any deceptive fighting maneuvers.

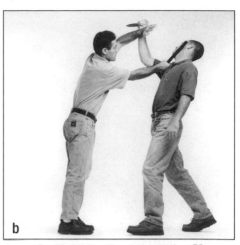

b

An option that was discussed earlier: You can use your free hand for the defense, and as soon as possible, counterattack with the stick.

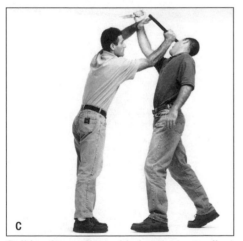

c

Striking the assailant with the rear (protruding) end of a short stick.

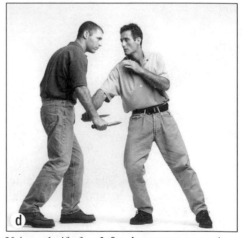

d

Using a knife for **defensive** purposes against an attacker stabbing with a knife. All techniques will be similar to those presented here.

Note: By **concealing your improvised weapon from the assailant's view**, you are ready for the adversary without allowing him to perceive what is about to happen. However, if you **reveal your weapon**, especially if it is a knife, while exhibiting a high degree of self-confidence and aggressiveness, you may be able to intimidate the assailant and sometimes even prevent the confrontation entirely. Your choice of behavioral tactics will depend on the situation and on your own nature.

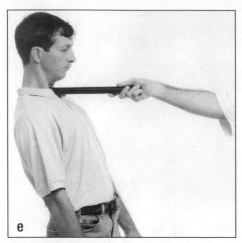

A stabbing attack with the stick.

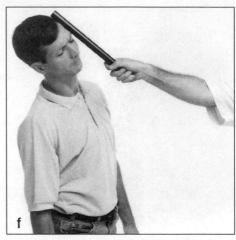

A striking attack (swing) to the assailant's head.

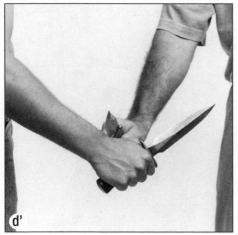

Close-up, photograph d: The defender's knife meets the attacker's wrist, in order to stop the stab more effectively.

Stick against Stick

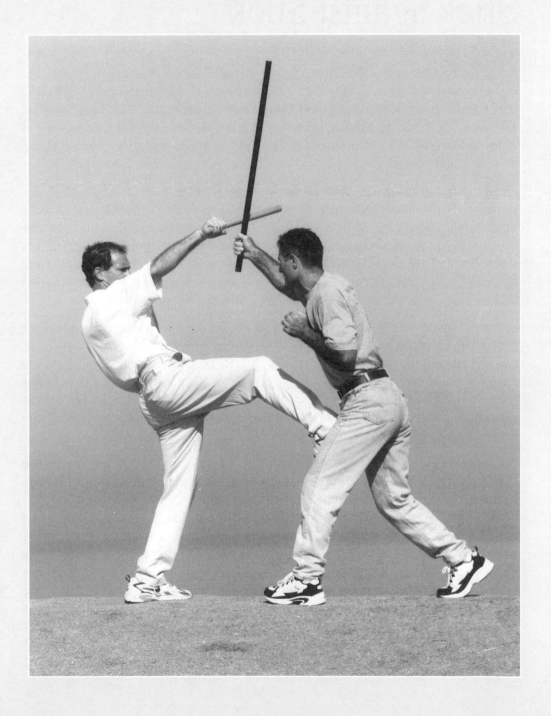

Chapter 9

Stick against Stick

Some martial arts specialize in the use of a straight or sword-shaped stick as the main weapon for defense and attack. These include the Japanese methods **Kendo** and **Kenjitsu**, the English method **Long-pole Fighters**, the Philippine method **Escrima** (or **Arnis de Mano**), branches of **Kung-Fu** and the Chinese method of fighting **Wu-Shu**, which employs a wide variety of spears and sticks, certain Indian methods, and others.

Even in the early stages of self-defense training, you must also learn the basic use of the stick in defense and attack, in order to protect yourself from injury, as sticks or stick-like objects are easily found in almost any environment where a fight may occur. There are advantages and disadvantages of each stick attack and defense, from different angles and under different conditions. For our purpose, the different modes of attack that are described in this chapter simulate not just stick attacks, but attacks that utilize weapons such as **an ax, a spear, a bayoneted rifle**, etc.

When it comes to self-defense, learning to use the stick against a knife attack, or against an unarmed assailant, is just as important as learning to use it against an assailant armed with a stick. Against knife attack, when armed with a stick, you can apply various techniques and defensive principles from those learned in defenses with stick against stick, in defenses with a short stick against a knife (see the previous chapter), and of course, the basic hand defenses that apply to dealing with an assailant armed with an edged weapon.

It is only natural for an armed fighter to focus his attention on his weapon and on that of his opponent. It is our hope that you will succeed in **freeing yourself from this limiting focus of attention**! You should be able to divide your attention, alert to all pertinent information that may increase your ability to react and function at a higher level. One must take notice, not only of the actions taken by the adversary with his weapon, but also of the actions he takes with other parts of his body. Be more aware of the measures you must take in defense or attack with your own weapon and with all the tools you possess on your body, i.e., your hands and legs. However, when you cannot use your stick, or when it hinders your potential, you should know when to stop using it in order to take more effective action with your hands and legs.

As in previous subjects, the basic principles of action and reaction underlying the defense techniques are identical and valid. (See Chap. 11: **Principles behind the Defense Techniques**.) Here too, there are active defense measures in which the weapon serves as an accessory, and there are evasive actions and body defenses, in which you distance yourself from the zone or line of danger.

Optional evasive body actions

Moving out of the range of attack; bursting forward to meet an attack before it has accumulated speed and force; moving out of the line of attack (whether the attack is vertical, horizontal, or otherwise); moving the body in the original direction of the attack (especially against a horizontal swing from the side) which weakens the attack's impact and delays or prevents its landing on the defender. You should use a combination of these movements along with the specific defenses using the stick.

Active defenses using the stick

- **Blocking**: Against swings, the defending stick hits the attacking stick at a right angle and stops it.

- **Sliding**: The defending stick is sent at an acute angle, in order to meet the attacking object (stick) and causing it to slide and be redirected to another course, which does not endanger the defender.

- **Deflecting**: Usually against stabbing attack, deflect the stabbing stick by a movement similar to that used in the inside or outside forearm defense against a straight punch or a straight knife stab.

When holding and using the stick, mainly for defensive actions, you can hold it in one hand only, or, if you prefer, in both hands.

When protecting a certain area of your body, you can usually hold the stick in two ways: (1) By turning your forearm (of the dominant hand) and the stick in **the same** direction, with the thumb or palm of your hand facing upwards, as shown in the technique *Basic Outside Defenses with a Stick*, photographs 2-4 and 8 (see next page). (2) By turning your forearm (of the dominant hand) and the stick in **opposite** directions, as in *Basic Outside Defenses with a Stick*, photographs 5-6 and 9-10.

Basic Outside Defenses with a Stick (against Circular Attacks)

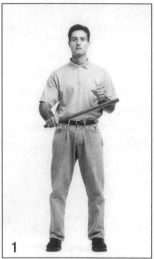

1

Outlet stance used for the basic **learning stage**: Standing with your legs slightly apart (passive stance), hold the stick in one or both hands. From this starting position you will proceed with each of the following defenses.

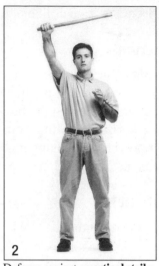

2

Defense against a **vertical strike from above**. One of the basic defenses where you send your stick in the direction of the attack, meeting the attacking stick (usually at a 90° angle).

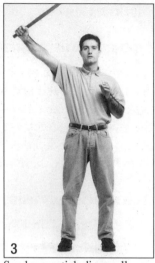

3

Send your stick diagonally upwards and to the side, to meet a **diagonal downward** strike directed towards the area of your head or shoulders.

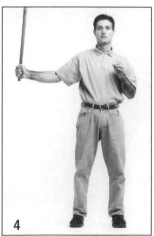

4

Send your stick to the side, in defense against a **horizontal swing** directed to head level or at medium height.

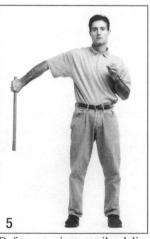

5

Defense against a strike delivered at **low or medium height**.

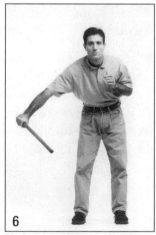

6

Defense against a strike delivered **diagonally upward** towards your body.

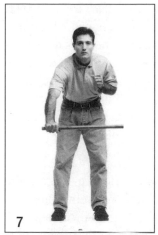

7

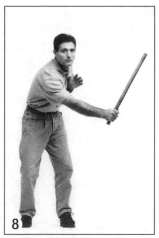

8

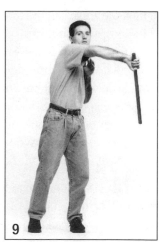

9

Defense against a **vertical strike from below**. Bend your upper body forward.

Photograph 8: Defense against a **diagonal upward** strike. Send the stick diagonally across your body. In all such techniques,

turn your body to enable a strong defense with the stick. The combination of raising the stick to a higher level (holding: thumb up) and a straight body, is an appropriate defense against a horizontal strike.

Defense against a **horizontal** attack to medium height. This time, hold the stick with your thumb facing down.

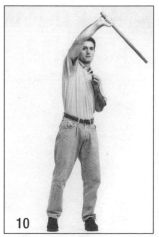

10

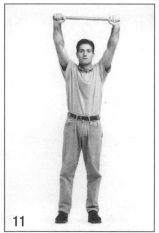

11

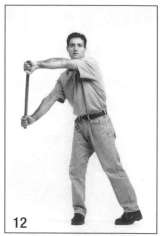

12

Defense against a **diagonal downward** strike directed towards your head or shoulders.

Another option for defending against a **vertical strike from above**. This time, you hold the stick in both hands. If you have to defend yourself against a sudden strike, you should bend your knees and drop your head down and slightly forward.

Another example of defense against a **horizontal swing from the side**. Hold the stick in both hands. In this defense, the right hand can be held higher and the left lower, or vice versa.

These defenses are based on a set of hand techniques called *360° Outside Defenses*. These are natural and reflexive techniques that serve as the basic set of outside defenses in the Krav Maga system. These outside defenses generally deal with attacks coming at the defender from the outer perimeter of an imaginary circle. You can hold the stick in one or both hands and use it for defense against different attacks, especially stick attacks. In all the basic defenses shown above, the defending stick meets the attacking stick and blocks it, at approximately a right (90°) angle. In later techniques, we will demonstrate the use of these basic defenses combined with body defenses and counterattacks.

Against a **sudden attacks** in particular, the defense will be reflexive. During the initial learning stage you will practice the defensive movement by itself. Later, one student will attack and the other defend. This will allow you to gain proficiency in the movement, learn to observe and understand the assailant's actions, as well as acquire good senses and skills in using the stick (which is, in effect, serving as an "extension" of your arm).

Caution: For safety reasons, during training and practice, always wear protective covering on the backs of your hands, and use unbreakable, unbendable sticks with no cracks or flaws.

Vertical Swing Downwards – Defending Stick Held in One Hand

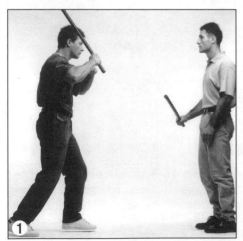
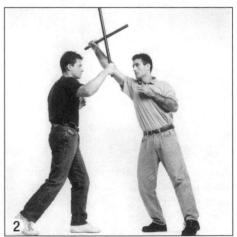

Begin from a proper starting stance, e.g., passive stance or with one foot (right) slightly forward.
Photograph 2: Send the stick forcefully to a horizontal (or diagonal) position, in order for the defense to block the opponent's attack.

Hold the stick in one hand, allowing the attacking stick to slide a short distance along your stick. The defensive hand movement with the stick "pulls" you into a body turn and a diagonal forward advance.

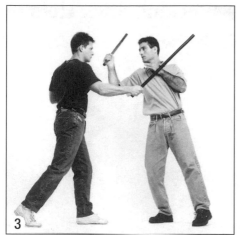

After excuting the defense, continue it with a rotating movement of your wrist, to bring the stick to a convenient position for an early and powerful counterattack.

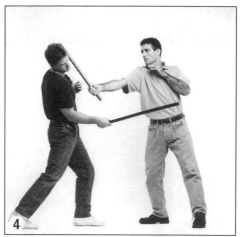

Continue the movement with a strike to the assailant's head. You can hit him at any angle between the horizontal and the vertical one. If you prefer, you can attack first with a strike to a less vulnerable target on the opponent's body.

The defending stick should meet the attacking stick **at least** in the middle and possibly even closer to the grip, so that the latter will not be able to slide and continue to hit you.

Your stick is extended forcefully towards the attacking stick, and should be held either horizontally or at a slightly downward angle away from your hand. During the defense, the attacking stick slides down a short distance along the defending stick and away from your hand. If the stick's original position was horizontal, the strike from the attacking stick should cause it to tilt downwards.

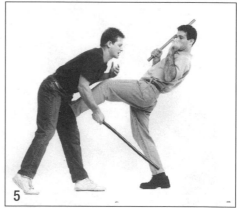

If needed, continue the action by delivering a second attack such as a kick to the assailant's groin, or move away from the scene of danger.

The counterattack with the stick may be a **whipping strike**, aimed to hurt the assailant in the forehead and brow area, or a **slashing swing**, in which the stick hits the target forcefully and then continues past it. It is also possible to use the stick to attack other, less vulnerable parts of the assailant's body (such as limbs, clavicle, shoulders, etc.), if you do not wish to cause him (or her) severe harm.

The body defense is performed with a diagonal step forward and sideways, and a body turn, by which you move out of the line of attack aimed at your head.

Vertical Strike Downwards – Blocking Stick Held in Both Hands, Counterattack by Kicking

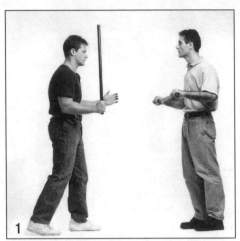

1

Hold the stick in two hands. One foot (the right) is slightly forward.

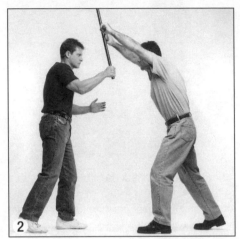

2

Block the attack, holding your stick in both hands and dropping your head between your shoulders. In addition to blocking the attack, and depending on the distance between you and your adversary, advance and shift your weight forward. This will prepare you to launch effective counterattacks.

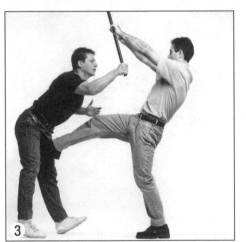

3

Execute your first counterattack: in this case, a kick to the groin. You can also attack with the stick, holding and rotating it in one hand, as shown in the previous technique.

In general, here you can also perform the previous technique at some time during the defensive action, but the stick is held in two hands, and you execute a body defense. In this technique, you move **forward** instead of **sideways**. Execute a strong defense against the attack from above, and advance, shifting your weight forward.

To reduce the shock created by blocking the attack, you should meet the attacking stick relatively close to the hand holding it. If the attack took you by surprise, it will be difficult for you to advance at the time indicated, and if the distance is great, you may find it difficult to execute a kicking attack. In either case, advance as early as possible or counterattack first with your stick.

While in the learning stage, you may feel more confident and comfortable in defending yourself against a stick attack by firmly grasping your stick at both ends. When performed properly, your defense should be able to block a forceful attack. In any case, your stick must be strong enough to withstand the force of the impact without breaking.

Note: In general, the more forceful the attack, the greater the need to execute the defense while holding the stick in both hands and to add a body defense.

If you fear a situation in which the **attacking weapon** may break, particularly if it is an ax, you must hold your head forward, between your shoulders. When the attack is less surprising, you should execute a greater body defense, moving diagonally forward with a slight body turn, as in the defense with one hand. (See the second technique described in this chapter.)

Horizontal Swing from the Side – Blocking Stick Held in One Hand

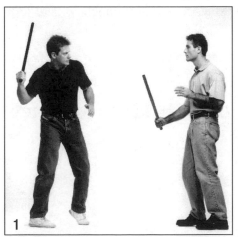

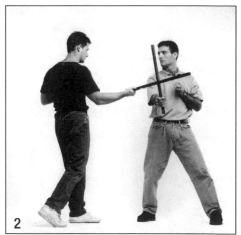

Start from an appropriate stance, e.g., with one foot (the right) in front.
Photograph 2: With a short, sharp defensive strike, send your stick to meet and block the

horizontal swing from the attacking stick. Execute a body turn and diagonal step forward. This helps to create a better angle for the defense and distances you from the focus of the attack.

Bounce the defending stick off the attacking stick in a short, sharp strike. This allows you to use your stick again as soon as possible to attack a vulnerable point on the assailant's body.

Here we demonstrate the principle of **keeping the aggressor from using his weapon again**, by grabbing it. However, this technique can also be performed

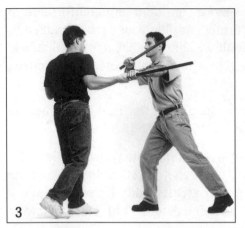

3

In a snappy movement, your stick "leaps" to the counterattack. As early as possible, grab the assailant's stick (or hand) so he will not be able to use it again.

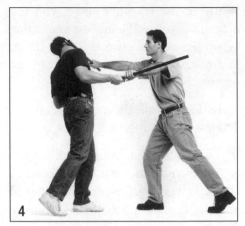

4

Execute an immediate attack to the assailant's head. *Variation: If you react fast enough, it is possible to kick your attacker at an earlier stage, simultaneously with your stick defense.*

without grabbing the attacking stick or the hand holding it. In this case, continue with counterattacks as necessary, with your stick, free hand (punches), and legs (kicks), or any combination thereof.

Variation: Execute the defense with the defending stick directed downwards and your hand positioned above it.

Horizontal Swing – Blocking Stick is Held in Two Hands

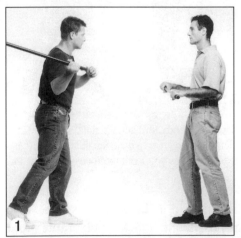

1

Hold the stick in two hands, while standing with legs slightly apart or with one leg slightly forward. The attack comes from your left.

This is another example of defense with a stick, in which you block the attack while holding the stick in both hands. Your stick should be sturdy enough to withstand the impact of the assailant's stick.

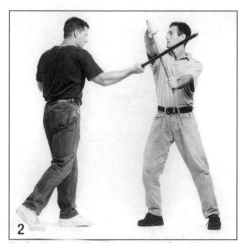

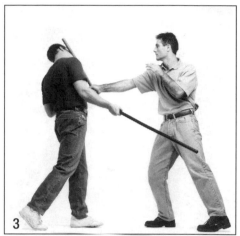

Defend yourself with a quick action. Block the attack by sending your stick diagonally sideways, while at the same time executing a body defense composed of a body turn and stepping (on your right foot) diagonally forward. Your elbows are almost straight.

"Bounce" the stick back from the block to the counterattack, releasing your lower hand's hold on your stick. As needed, attack the assailant's head or any other appropriate, vulnerable point. Continue as necessary, executing further attacks with the stick, or using kicks or punches.

As in all the techniques that have been previously described, the defense action with the stick, together with the body turn and the diagonal forward advance, have made it possible to stop the attacker's stick approximately at its center and slightly closer to the hand that is holding it. Be sure to avoid a defense that only stops the hand holding the stick, since **the stick will continue to strike**. Likewise, take care not to stop the stick at its far end, as it is liable to slide on your stick and come back at you.

Note: In essence, **all of the techniques demonstrated so far are similar**, since they use a blocking defense against different types of swinging attacks that are aimed at your body from the outside in.

Straight Stab – Deflecting by Inside Defense

The angle of your position relative to that of the attacker, as well as the position of your stick, dictate the type of defense and the nature of the counterattack that you will use. In the inside defense movement, your stick delivers a fast, sharp strike to the assailant's stick, deflects it, and is then "launched" from the assailant's stick directly into a counterattack. To enable an effective deflection, the lower part of your stick must be lower than the front of the assailant's stick, and the higher part of your stick should be higher than his stick.

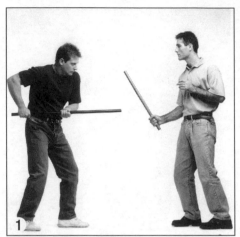

1

In this case, you are in a starting position that demands an inside defense against the forthcoming straight attack.

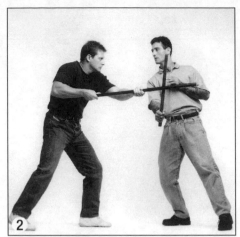

2

Apply an inside defense, deflecting the stab in a sharp, explosive movement. At the same time, execute a body defense by turning slightly and stepping diagonally forward. As it is difficult to determine the height of the stab, defend with your stick held more vertically, so as to protect a larger area of your body.

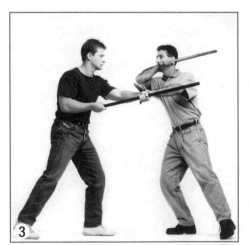

3

As you are preparing to deliver an immediate counterattack, send your other hand to grab the attacking weapon.

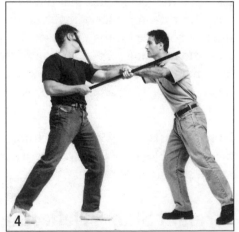

4

Counterattack your opponent immediately. You can execute additional attacks with the stick or attack with punches or kicks, according to the circumstances.

Possible initial counterattacks: Stab with your stick, deliver a swinging strike with the stick, kick, punch with your free hand, or, if the assailant is at close range, strike with the rear part of the stick, the side that protrudes from your hand. To prevent the assailant from using his weapon again, you can grab the attacking stick or the hand holding it.

Straight Stab – Deflecting by Outside Defense

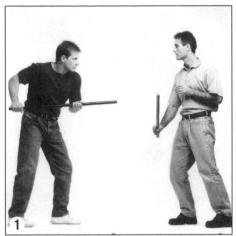

In this instance, you are starting from a position that necessitates an outside defense against the attack.

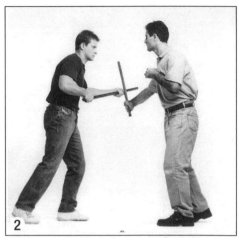

Apply the outside defense to deflect the attack with a fast, sharp movement. At the same time, perform a body defense by turning your body slightly and advancing with a diagonal step forward (with your rear leg).

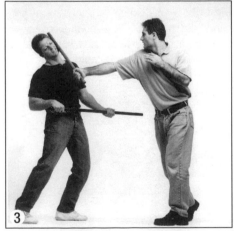

Execute your initial counterattack. You can then perform additional attacks, using your stick or delivering punches and kicks, as dictated by the circumstances.

In order to practice this specific defense, stand and hold the stick across your body at an angle necessitating an outside defense. The manner in which the stick is held dictates that an outside defense is the fastest and most effective.

The first counterattack can be a strike with the stick to the assailant's head (from the outside inward), a stab at a vulnerable point on his head, or a kick to the groin.

If the attack is more of a **surprise**, you will still apply an outside defense. However, your other actions (i.e., body defenses and counterattacks) will probably come at a comparatively later stage. You should practice to minimize this delay!

Straight, Low Stab – Outside, Downward Defense

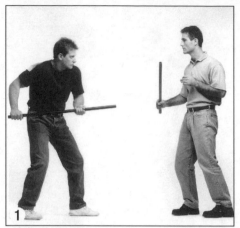

In this case, your stick is raised slightly. This starting position will necessitate an outside, downward defense technique against any type of low stabbing attack.

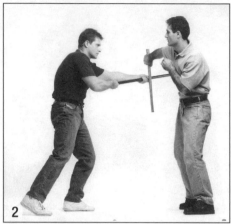

The assailant attacks with a low "stab". From your starting position, you execute an outside, downward defense with a sharp and fast movement, deflecting the attack to the side. This deflection "pulls" you into a body turn and forward diagonal advance, which forms your "body defense." These movements serve to create both a body defense and a better position from which to launch the counterattacks.

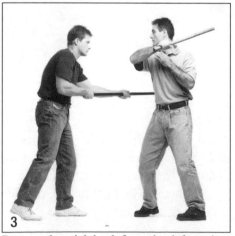

Bounce the stick back from the defense into your counterattack.

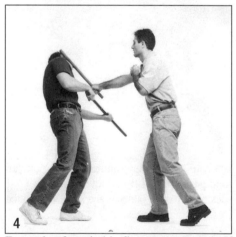

Example of a suitable first counterattack. If necessary, advance on your right foot to achieve the correct distance for striking the assailant.

With the aid of the stick, execute a downward, outward deflection. To make this action fast and powerful, lift your elbow and turn your hand, moving it aside, causing your stick to turn downward and deflect the attack, sideways.

Against a low stab, you can execute a regular inside or outside defense as previously described, but that is possible only if your stick is at the height of the stab, before it occurs. For this purpose, you must lower your stance and your hand, as in applying the principle demonstrated in the technique ***Stab, Straight Hold – Inside Defense from the Outside***. (See Chap. 1: **Defense against Knife Attack**.)

Basic Attack against Armed Assailant – Strike with Stick and Kick

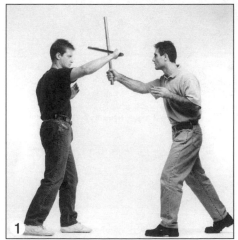

Attack forcefully with your stick, advancing as needed and shifting your weight forward. As expected, your opponent executes a defense against this attack.

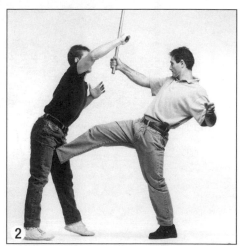

Proceed to attack, using a regular kick that is directed to the adversary's groin, and delivered when he is concentrating on protecting himself from the stick attack.

Here, we demonstrate a fast, simple, and highly effective technique as a tactical attack against an assailant armed with a stick. In a confrontation in which both you and your opponent are armed with sticks, you can apply such a technique in order to overpower him, even if you are not an expert in using a stick.

The technique is based on two attacks, which are executed in **broken or staggered rhythm**, i.e., the second attack, is sent before the first one is completed. The second attack will hit the assailant, even if the first one merely distracted his attention. For this purpose, you can use the following combinations: (1) Attacking by kicking, which serves as a deception, and then attack with the stick. (2) Charging with several stick attacks combined with kicks. (3) First throwing something at the assailant and then following with a stick attack, etc.

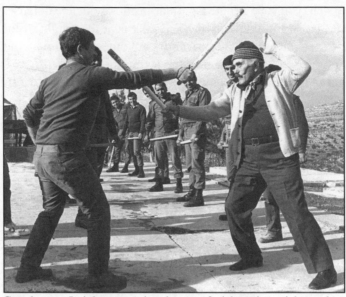

Grandmaster Imi demonstrating the use of stick against stick attack.

Defense against Two Armed Assailants

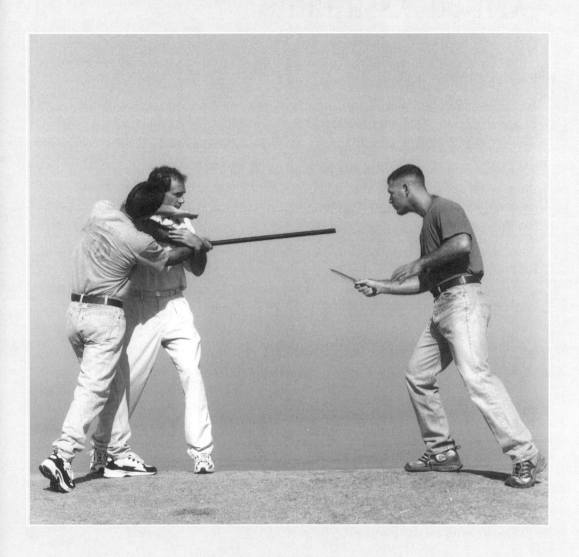

Chapter 10

Defense against Two Armed Assailants

When facing an opponent, you should find out as soon as possible whether there is **another attacker** that may endanger you as it entirely changes the situation.

A confrontation with two or more assailants can assume the nature of a **fight**, a **self-defense** scenario, or a **combination** of the two. Under such conditions, some of the tactics that you apply will be different from those employed against a single opponent.

From the moment you realize that you are facing more than one attacker, it is imperative to expand your attention, so as not to miss an important move made by **any** of the combatants. You must put yourself in the best possible position, relative to all the assailants.

Note: If you devote too much of your attention to one assailant, **the other(s) will be free to act undisturbed**. This is analogous to a confrontation with a single assailant, when one focuses solely on the attacker's hands, for example, leaving oneself vulnerable to the attacker's kicks. This, of course, should never be done!

In this chapter, we will consider the confrontation as a self-defense incident in which you are facing two assailants, in this case armed ones. We will present and analyze a typical example in which one attacker is holding a knife and the other, a stick. In order to simplify the presentation and understanding of the subject, let us assume throughout the entire chapter that each assailant is attacking in a specific and defined manner. From this particular example, we can learn and deduce many valuable principles:

- The situation is extremely dangerous. Therefore, if possible, **leave the area as soon as you can**.

- Whenever possible, you should **take the initiative and make the first move**. Do not wait for the assailant(s) to start.

- **Avoid devoting excessive attention to one assailant only**. You should first neutralize one of your opponents as quickly and effectively as possible, and then deal with the other(s) as necessary.

- **Decrease your distance from one assailant**, in order to defend and attack effectively. Do this in such a way that it puts you farther away from the other aggressor(s), to enhance your safety.

- **Avoid standing or passing between the two attackers**. If you cannot avoid passing between them, do it as quickly as you can. If possible or when necessary, make your move while taking action against the more dangerous assailant, or against both of them.

- Take action both to defend yourself and to attack the aggressors, by placing yourself so that **one attacker serves as a shield, or barrier, between you and the other(s)**. This can be achieved by moving in the correct direction or by turning and positioning one assailant in the appropriate place, between you and the other assailant(s).

- **Shoving one assailant towards the other**, especially after the first has been forcefully counterattacked, will give you an instant advantage by creating a significant disturbance to the actions of the second assailant. Take advantage of this in order to neutralize one or both assailants, or immediately seize the opportunity for a self-controlled retreat from the scene of the incident.

- In an asymmetrical situation, when each assailant is carrying a different kind of weapon, each of which poses a different level of strength and threat, you should first take the action that **limits the attack capability of the more dangerous aggressor**, while taking into account the possibility of any further action from all the assailants.

  For example: In terms of the effectiveness of one type of weapon versus another, at first, when the assailants are relatively far from the defender, **the stick is usually more dangerous than the knife** because of its comparatively longer reach. Therefore, in most such situations, the first action should be taken against the assailant holding the stick, even if he is not the one who made the first move to attack! In addition, the stick can be taken from and utilized against the other assailant (the one armed with a knife).

- In asymmetrical situations where one assailant is armed with a knife and the other with a stick, apply defensive measures against the one holding the knife, **only if he has momentarily become the more dangerous assailant**, e.g., if he has moved within close range and has attacked you by surprise. In most cases, even if the knife-wielding assailant is closer to you, it is possible (and recommended) to "escape" towards the one with the stick, and attack him.

- Whenever possible, **disarm one assailant and use his weapon for defense and counterattack**. For example, the stick will be an effective weapon against the knife, but the opposite is not necessarily true!

Beware: Both weapons must not fall into the hands of a single assailant.

In practicing the following defense techniques against two or more assailants, first apply the principles detailed above, under clearly defined conditions. Then practice **variations** in which the attackers are armed with the same or different weapons, or are using different techniques to attack you while they approach you from opposite directions. You can also simulate other realistic situations, e.g., on a stairway, while sitting down, in confined areas or with limited lighting, etc.

This will enable you to turn the unusual into the usual, the strange and unfamiliar into the familiar. In this way you train to improvise, and in time of need, you will have the skill to apply the correct response to a new problem. **This is the key to improving your ability to deal effectively with real-life situations**.

Two Assailants – One on the Right, Armed with a Stick and the Other on the Left, with a Knife

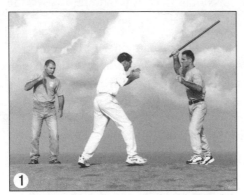

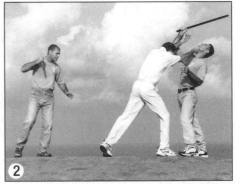

Starting position. The assailant with the stick is diagonally to your right, and the one with the knife is diagonally to your left. Both are attacking you. If possible, **take the initiative** and do not wait for your opponents. Attack one of them (preferably the assailant armed with the stick), using the proper technique.

Employ the defense and counterattack against the assailant armed with the stick. In this example he is attacking you with an overhead swing. The knife-wielding assailant must now change his line of attack, and the safety distance between you and him has increased.

Assume that the assailants are approximately equidistant from you. The assailant with the stick poses the greater danger because of the longer reach of his weapon: he can reach you faster due to this advantage.

Based on the principle of executing defenses and attacks according to the level of risk posed by each assailant, **the first action will usually be taken against the assailant with the stick**. An exception to this rule exists, of course, when the knife-wielding assailant has stabbed at you by surprise or is at a very close range. In this

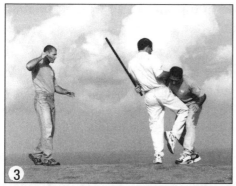

As the second attacker has been surprised, you can continue now by grabbing the first assailant (step with your left foot) and counterattacking him with a knee to the groin.

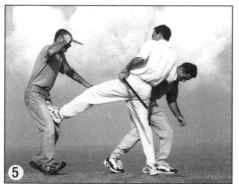

At the proper range, stop the knife-wielding assailant with a kick to the groin.

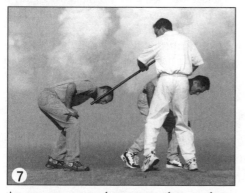

As necessary, use the weapon that you have taken to counterattack.

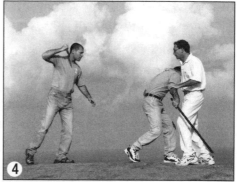

Step with your right foot to rotate the stick-wielding assailant. He will serve as a barrier between you and the second assailant (the one with the knife). **Beware**: The knife-wielding attacker will invariably attempt to go around or over the "barrier" in order to attack you.

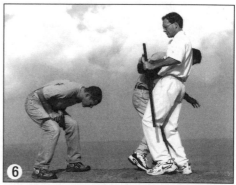

If the stick is still in the hands of the first attacker, use a leverage technique to take the stick from the assailant's hands. (If needed, do this with the help of your knee or thigh.)

case, you have no other choice but to take first action against him, as shown later in this chapter in the technique *Two Assailants - First Action against the Knife-Wielding Assailant*.

In the example pictured above, the defense technique is applied against the assailant holding the stick. The actions of advancing towards the first aggressor and turning him so as to obstruct the second, are executed **at top speed and without turning your back completely on the second assailant**.

In this example, you had enough time to disarm the first attacker. This you do by rotating the stick in the attacker's hand, bringing the stick close to his forearm. In other cases, the weapon may fall to the ground as a result of the counterattacks, or you may not have enough time to take the weapon, rather just a split second to jump backwards, or you may have to act immediately against the second assailant, using "only" your hands and legs.

Two Assailants – One on the Right, Armed with a Knife and the Other on the Left, with a Stick

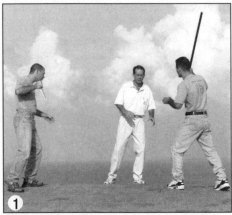

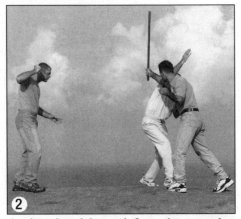

Starting position: You are attacked by two armed men; on your right there is an assailant armed with a knife, and on your left an assailant armed with a stick.

Against the stick attack from above, apply a stabbing defense technique to the outside of the attacking forearm, while bursting forward preferably on the same foot as the defending hand. This particular move also enables you to easily perform the next stage, and increases your distance from the second attacker.

Here too, we see how the basic principles are applied. The defense technique is a stabbing defense to the outside of the attack, that enables you to go behind the aggressor without passing between the two attackers, and **without turning your back on the one with the knife**. In this example, as well as in the first, you succeed in disarming the initial assailant, though only at a later stage (as compared to the first example above). **Other possible scenarios**: The stick may fall from the first attacker's hands, as a result of the counterattacks, or you may not have enough time to disarm him before having to foil the actions of the second assailant.

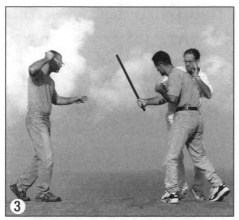

3 Continue with another step, in order to move behind the first assailant.

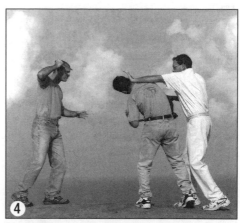

4 Simultaneously, counterattack and step behind this assailant. Your move forces the assailant with the knife to change his line of attack.

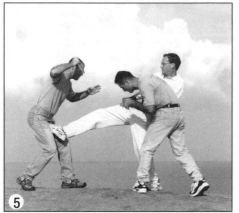

5 Kick the second assailant in order to stop him at a distance.

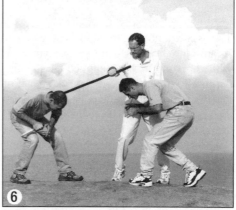

6 When the situation permits, disarm the first assailant and use his weapon as necessary.

Note: The first two techniques only partially demonstrate how to place the first assailant in front of the other one.

Caution: If one of the assailants drops his weapon, you should **prevent the other from grabbing it and having two weapons** at his disposal!

Two Assailants – How to Move in order to Increase Your Distance from the Second Assailant

First option:

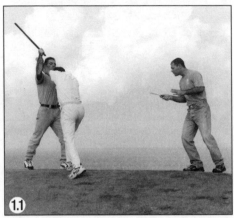

The assailant holding the stick is on your left. Against the stick attack from above, you have, while bursting forward, applied the stabbing defense to the inside of the attack, an action that does not place you far enough away from the second assailant. This technique includes a counterattack. Since you are defending with your left hand and your right leg is in front, you will continue as follows:

The following 3 sets of photographs demonstrate the different options that the defender has for turning the first assailant towards the second. This became necessary when your first action failed to place you far enough away from the threat posed by the second assailant. In the previous technique you succeeded in moving behind the first attacker (the one holding the stick) in your first defensive action. In the case presented here, you did not.

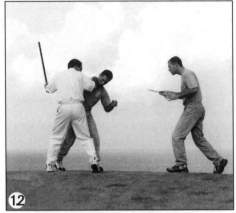

Turn the first assailant in an outward motion, by taking a diagonal step forward with your rear (left) leg.

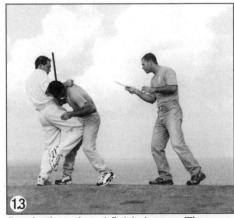

Step backwards and finish the turn. Thus, you will increase your distance from the second assailant and position the first one as a barrier between the two of you. Now execute an additional counterattack against the first assailant.

The type of attack executed by the first assailant and the position of your legs when executing the initial defense technique, combined with the angle and distance from the second assailant, are the factors that largely determine the direction of the turn.

Second option:

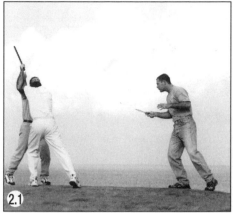

The assailant holding the stick is on your left. Against the stick attack from above, you have applied the stabbing defense to the inside of the attack with your left hand, putting you even farther from the other assailant. The technique also includes a counterattack. Here, your front (left) leg is the same as your defending (also left) hand.

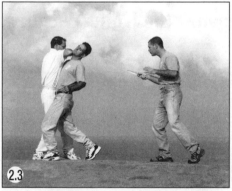

The first assailant is now forming a barrier to the second. Continue with counterattacks or distance yourself rapidly from the danger zone.

With your second step, turn the stick-wielding assailant **to your left**, having executed the defense with your left foot forward (photographs 2.1–2.3), or **to your right**, when you have executed a defense with your right foot forward

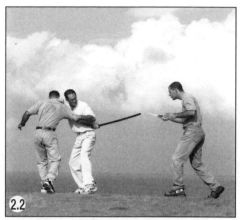

Proceed in a continuous movement. Because you have put your left leg forward, take a step forward with your rear (right) foot, and then turn. This move can be done only if **the second assailant is relatively far away**, since during the turn you will have your back to him, which is definitely an undesirable situation on your part. Pass between the two aggressors as fast as possible, execute the turn, and position the first assailant as a shield between you and the second one.

Third option:

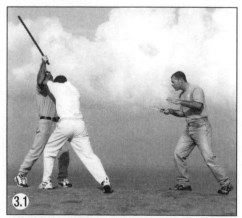

As in the previous set, you have executed the technique with your left leg forward, but here, due to lack of time and space, you cannot pass between the two assailants.

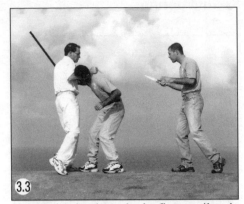

Continue with a small step onto your left leg. Turn and step back with your right leg, forcefully turning the stick-wielding assailant.

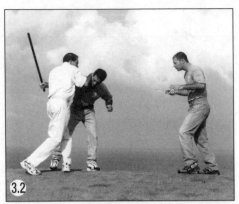

Your action has brought the first assailant in front of you, blocking the way of the knife-wielding assailant. Proceed as necessary.

(photographs 1.1–1.3), or **with your left leg** forward in case you did not have sufficient space and time to pass between the two assailants (photographs 3.1–3.3).

Note: If the second assailant closes in on you from behind and poses an immediate danger while you are applying the defense technique against the first, you can hurt him and stop his advance, for example with a **defensive back kick** (a straight kick backwards), and then proceed with your actions against the first attacker.

Two Assailants – First Action against the Knife-Wielding Assailant

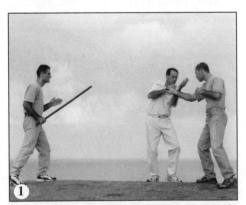

The knife-wielding assailant is on your left, and the attacker with the stick is on your right. Execute an inside defense technique (from the outside) against the assailant holding the knife, who is attacking you at relatively close range, and possibly by surprise, using a straight stab.

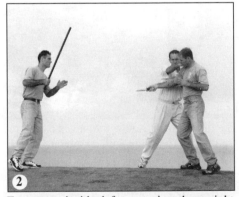

Execute an inside defense against the straight attack with the knife, and deliver a counterattack while moving diagonally forward.

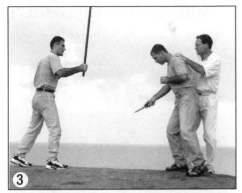

3

Being aware of the actions of the other assailant, maintain control over the first knife-wielding attacker and move further behind him.

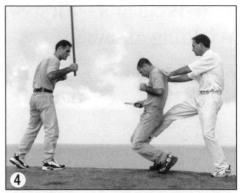

4

Move behind the assailant and deliver a stomping kick to the back of his knee, pushing him forward. The second attacker's path is now blocked.

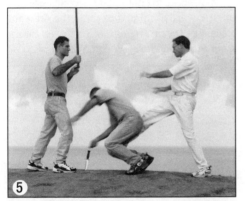

5

As you shove the first aggressor towards the other, he creates an obstacle. He will invariably block the second assailant's path, or at least may interfere with his ability to reach you in the shortest, most direct line.

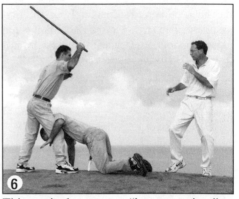

6

This tactical maneuver "buys you time" to continue your counterattack, defend as needed, or move away.

You have been surprised by a stabbing attempt at close range, and must take action against the stab and the attacker. If the assailant with the stick is relatively far away, as in the photograph, you may have enough time to execute counterattacks and take other measures against the first, knife-wielding assailant. If you are pressed for time, you can still execute a defense and possibly even deliver one counterattack to the knife-wielding assailant.

Remember: You must **immediately thereafter engage the attacker armed with the stick**, or jump backwards to gain distance from both assailants.

If you have disarmed the knife-wielding assailant, you can use the knife for your counterattacks and may even consider throwing it at the second assailant (if you know how) to stop him from attacking, and then burst forward to attack him.

Two Assailants – First Short Action against the Knife-Wielding Assailant

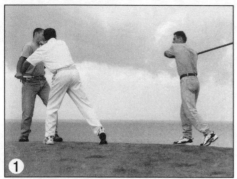

Block the oriental (upward) knife-stab, which has been delivered surprisingly by the first assailant. The stick-wielding assailant is too close. Your options may be to jump backwards or burst (sideways) towards him.

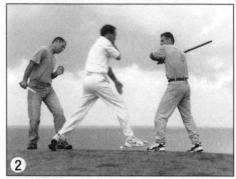

As you choose to confront the second assailant, burst towards him and execute the relevant technique: *Defense against a Horizontal Swing from the Side (Baseball Bat Swing)*.

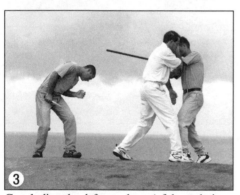

Concluding the defense phase (of the technique against a horizontal swing with a stick).

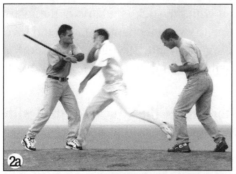

Photograph 2, taken from the front: Bursting against the second assailant.

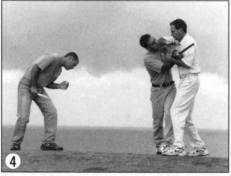

The counterattack against the second assailant is executed as you position him between you and the other one, to block the way of the knife-wielding assailant. At all times you should be aware of the actions taken by the other attacker.

When left without enough time to deal with the knife-wielding assailant who attacks you by surprise at a relatively close range, you need to execute a suitable defense and simultaneously counterattack him. You should then spring immediately towards the second assailant, minimizing the distance between you and him, thus rendering his stick attack ineffective.

Chapter 11

Principles behind the Defense Techniques

In this chapter we will deal with various principles that are the fundamentals of defensive actions. These principles apply to defending against hand attacks (all sorts of punches or stabbing movements), leg and foot attacks, or attacks involving the use of weapons. The general purpose of a defensive action is to **hinder the attack**, preventing the assailant from striking the target. In addition, a properly executed technique should enable the defender to deliver an effective and immediate counterattack or prepare the way for a controlled retreat.

The self-defense techniques form a significant part of the Krav Maga system. They are much more than just a random collection of useful techniques. Each of them can be taken apart and analyzed methodically. This helps to break down each technique into its basic components and understand the general underlying principles. The principles addressed in this section are divided according to these common components that serve to create the earliest, shortest and most effective defensive response to an attack. By knowing, understanding, and internalizing these principles, you will be able to **react with the correct responses to the incident you are facing, and deal much more efficiently with real situations**, some of which you never encountered in training. Training according to these principles, practicing against variations in the attack, and learning to critically examine danger and problem-solving, will definitely prepare you more effectively to deal with real violent confrontations.

Body Defense (Evasion)

The term **evasion** or **body defense** refers to moving the target, so that the attack, whether it is a punch, a kick, or an attack with a weapon, will not "hit home." The basic evasions are the following:

Horizontal Body Movements
1. **Moving away, retreating**: In this defense, you move out of range of the attack. Your movement is along an imaginary line between you and the aggressor. You

can either move away entirely, i.e., retreating by one or more steps, or you can move the area of the body targeted for attack backwards, e.g., bend your upper body back, which moves your head and neck out of reach of a punch or a knife slash.

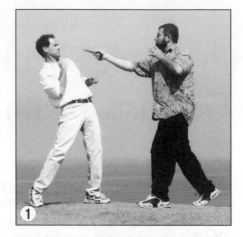

2. **Reducing the distance with a forward advance**: In this action, you close the gap between yourself and the assailant, so that weapons or limbs attacking you from the outside, e.g., a foot executing a roundhouse kick or the end of a stick in a horizontal strike from the side, will not hit the target with their fast-moving, more dangerous parts, which are the areas furthest from their axes of movement. The part that hits you will be, at worst, the part nearest to the source of movement and the base of the attacking weapon or limb.

Remember: This defense alone will usually **not suffice against straight attacks**. However, if the body defense is executed correctly and with proper timing, even the adversary's straight attack will not have enough time to cover a long distance and achieve high speed, and it will thus lack enough momentum and be rendered much less effective. In Krav Maga, most of the techniques that apply this principle also utilize a suitable defensive hand technique as an integral part of the overall defense.

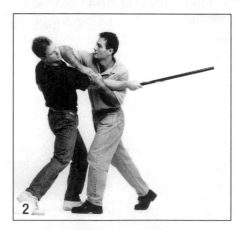

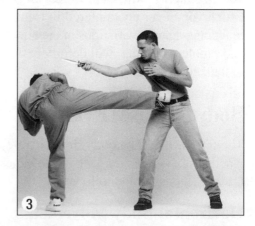

3. **Sideways movement**: Here, you move along an imaginary line perpendicular to the line between you and the aggressor. This defense is usually accompanied by a **body turn** (to be explained later). As a result of this movement, an attack directed straight ahead will go **past you** rather than **hit you**. Even if the attack is executed

in a circling or roundhouse movement, the correct evasion will take you out of the effective range of attack and minimize its impact, though in this case you will usually have to move a longer distance.

The following drawings show defenses by a body movement to the side (view from above). The attached legend applies to all the drawings in this chapter.

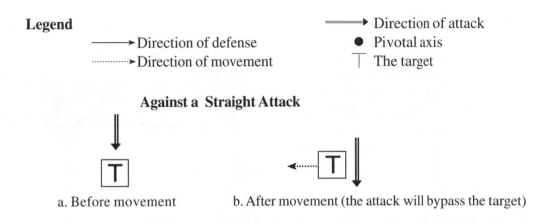

Legend
→ Direction of defense
⋯► Direction of movement
⟹ Direction of attack
● Pivotal axis
⊤ The target

Against a Straight Attack

a. Before movement   b. After movement (the attack will bypass the target)

Against a Roundhouse Attack

a. Before movement   b. Sideways movement (creates a reduced impact)

Body Turn

In this action, you move along a vertical axis, similar to the way a door moves on its hinges. When the attacks are in a straight movement, correct location of the axis will ensure an effective body defense, away from the line of attack. Although this defense by itself will not be entirely sufficient against attacks from the outside (roundhouse attacks), attacks that follow a long trajectory, it will definitely reduce their impact.

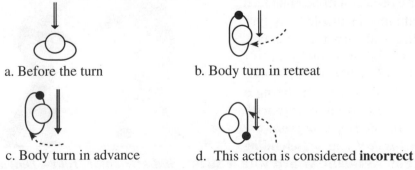

a. Before the turn   b. Body turn in retreat

c. Body turn in advance   d. This action is considered **incorrect**

Krav Maga's defense techniques usually include a body turn combined with the defender's advancing diagonally forward and to the side. This applies, for example, to *Threat from the Front, from a Distance* (in Chap. 4: **Neutralizing a Threat at Gunpoint**); *Stab, Straight Hold – Inside Defense from the Outside; Stab*, *Oriental Hold – Diagonal Forearm Defense* (in Chap. 1: **Defense against Knife Attack**); *Hand Defenses against Regular Kick*, and others.

Defense by Changing Height

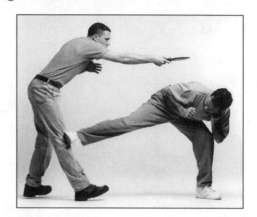

In this action you "change" your height, causing the attack to pass over or under your body. In Krav Maga, such defenses include **lowering your body** by bending the upper body and knees or **lifting the intended target**, e.g., raising your leg against a low kick aimed at your shin or knee, neutralizing the immediate danger to your leg.

Combining Several Principles in One Technique

For the body defenses to be effective, various forms of evasion are added and integrated. For example, see the following:

1. **Moving in "all" directions**, e.g., evasion by diagonal forward or backward movement. This is created by combining movements to the side with a forward or backward movement. In effect, we have eight main directions of horizontal movement (similar to the compass rose), not just the four lateral directions as described up to now. (The full range of possibilities is, of course, an infinite number of diagonal directions.)

2. **Combination of movement with a body turn**. In many of the Krav Maga techniques, the effectiveness of your evasions will be enhanced by combining a suitable body turn with diagonal forward advances. These techniques include, for example: *Threat from the Front, from a Distance* (**Neutralizing a Threat at Gunpoint**); *Stab with Stick – Inside Defense from the Outside/Inside* (Chap. 3: **Defending**

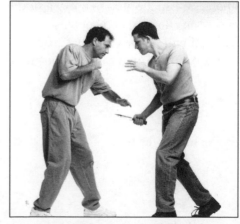

against an Assailant Armed with a Stick); *Stab, Oriental Hold – Diagonal*

Forearm Defense (Chap. 1: **Defense against Knife Attack**) and others.

3. **Combination of movement in the appropriate direction, with a change of height**, e.g., as demonstrated in *Stab, Straight Hold – Lateral Body Defense and Kick* (Chap. 1: **Defense against Knife Attack**). You move sideways and tilt your body downwards so as to move away and duck under the line of attack.

Hand or Foot Defenses

We will now discuss the principles of hand or leg movements in executing defense techniques. As previously explained, Krav Maga systematically combines the defenses performed by the different limbs, with a corresponding evasive body movement. Exceptions to this rule are sudden, reflexive defenses, such as *360° Outside Defenses*, when time constraints permit only sending a limb to block or deflect the attack. In such situations, it is sometimes more difficult to actually move the body for an effective evasive maneuver, and almost impossible to move the whole body, i.e., the center of gravity of the defender's body.

Direction of Limb Movement during the Defense

1. **Inside defenses**: In these actions, the defending limb operates from the outside to the inside, with your body as the reference point. For example, see: *Inside Defense from the "Live" Side* and *Inside Defense from the Outside* (Chap. 1: **Defense against Knife Attack/Knife in Straight Hold**).

2. **Outside defenses**: In these actions, the defending limb acts from the inside out; the reference point is your body. These techniques also include defenses in which the defending limb moves up or down from the center. (See techniques on forearm defenses against knife stab in oriental or regular holds in Chap. 1: **Defense against Knife Attack**.)

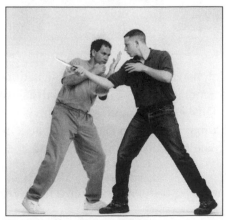

An example of Inside defense

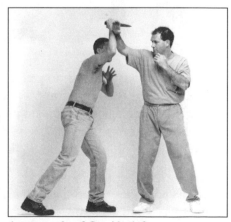

An example of Outside defense

Direction of Impact on Attacking Limb

Here we will discuss the direction and angle at which the attacking limb hits the defending limb, and vice versa. There are four different types and directions of impact.

1. **Vertical impact**: The first possibility is a vertical impact of the defending hand or foot on the attacking limb, e.g., against a straight knife stab or a punch. As a result, the attack is deflected from its original direction of movement. (See photograph a.) **Examples**: *Stab with Stick – Inside Defense from the Outside/Inside* (Chap. 3: **Defending against an Assailant Armed with a Stick**) where at the moment of contact, the palm moves inward only (as opposed to the sliding defense); *Straight Stab – Deflecting by Inside/Outside Defense* (Chap. 9: **Stick against Stick**).

   The second possibility is a vertical impact against the attacking limb moving in a rotating or roundhouse movement, with the objective of **stopping and blocking the attack**, as demonstrated in photograph b. See the following forearm defenses: *Sudden Stab from the Front – Oriental/Regular Hold* (Chap. 1: **Defense against Knife Attack**); *Overhead Swing – Stabbing Defense to the Inside of the Attack* (Chap. 3: **Defending against an Assailant Armed with a Stick**).

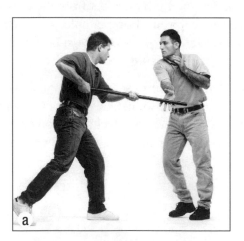 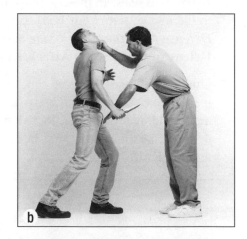

When the defender has no weapon for defensive purposes, a possible action for reducing the intensity of impact on the defending limb is **to stop the attack over a distance**, rather than at a single point. This action is analogous to the way that a shock absorber functions. The defender may also add a slant, to create a more acute angle of impact, and a sliding movement between the attacking and the defending limbs.

A more appropriate defense action against such a powerful attack, with a non-vertical impact, is a slant to create a sliding movement.

a. Defense whose impact deflects the attack, altering its course.
b. Blocking defense: stops the attack at a 90° angle.
c. In the case of a very powerful attack, a 90° block is not always recommended.

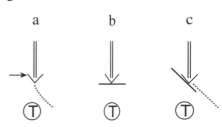

2. **Sliding**: This occurs when the defending limb goes out to deflect the attack and meets or hits the attacking limb at an acute angle.

Examples: *Overhead Swing – Stabbing Defense to the Inside /Outside of the Attack* (Chap.3: **Defending against an Assailant Armed with a Stick**), when the hand defense is referred to as a "stabbing defense."

In the techniques *Stab, Straight Hold – Inside Defense from the Outside* (Chapter 1: **Defense against Knife Attack**) and *Inside Sliding Defense against Straight Punch*, your hand (forearm) is sent diagonally forward to slide along and redirect the assailant's forearm and punch, away from the intended target. In the second technique, the sliding defense develops along the same line of movement into a punch delivered to the attacker.

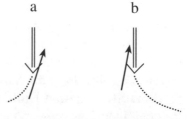

The direction from which the attacking limb (or object) is met by the defending limb.

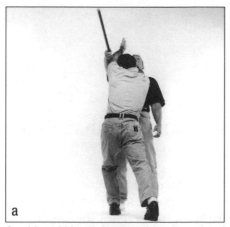

Outside stabbing defense against an overhead stick attack.

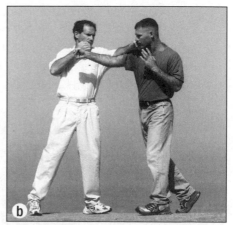

Inside sliding defense against straight punch, with an attack at the end of the defense.

3. **Accompanying or sweeping defenses**:
   In these actions, the defending limb
   gives a new direction to the attacking
   limb, in that it joins the attacking limb,
   while accompanying it and deflecting
   it from its original course. Though this
   principle is not often seen in Krav Maga,
   we can understand it from the technique:
   Threat from the Front, from a Distance
   (Chap. 4: **Neutralizing a Threat at
   Gunpoint**); or *Stab, Straight Hold –
   Inside Defense to the "Live" Side*.

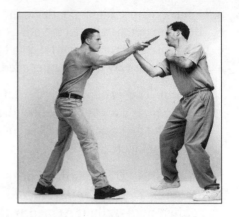

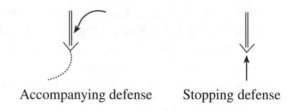

Accompanying defense   Stopping defense

4. **Stopping an attack with a counterattack**: Attack to the assailant's striking
   limb (or his body) while it is active, e.g.,
   Defense against Regular Stab (Chap.
   8: **Short Stick against Knife Attack**).
   You can launch a counterattack on the
   aggressor's body while he advances, as
   soon as he has achieved the proper range.
   Example: Kicking an assailant's body
   when he is attempting to stab you, used
   against any sort of knife attack.

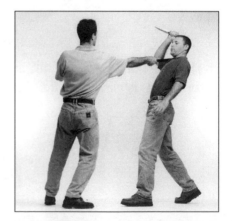

Combination of Body Actions and Limb Actions – Analysis of Different Techniques

Most defense techniques in Krav Maga apply a combination of certain body defense
principles with certain limb defense principles. Several techniques are analyzed
below. **Different defensive principles within a given technique should never
contradict one another**. This is a basic rule guiding the theory behind the Krav
Maga system.

1. *Inside Defense against Regular Kick*: While slightly bending your upper body forward, send your hand to meet the kicking leg (shin) and **deflect** it in an inside defense with **vertical impact**. Your body defense (evasion) is integrated into your hand movement and consists of two moves: a **body turn** and a forward **diagonal advance** to evade the line of attack. Although the full technique is not shown here, a defense based on the same theory is illustrated, though at a different height, in the defense against a stabbing attack with a stick (or bayonet).

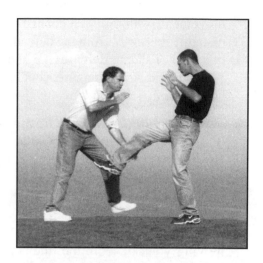

2. *Stab, Oriental Hold – Diagonal Forearm Defense* (Chapter 1: **Defense against Knife Attack**): Advance diagonally forward, with a quick inward turn that reinforces your body defense. In the forearm defense, you **stop** the attacking forearm and **block** it. Your elbow is below the assailant's in order to create a slight **outward sliding effect,** or more precisely, to prevent the attacking forearm from sliding inward towards your body.

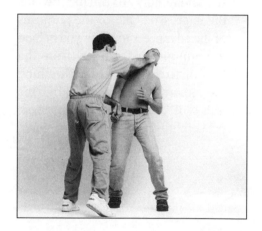

3. *Overhead Swing – Stabbing Defense to the Inside of the Attack* (Chap. 3: **Defending against an Assailant Armed with a stick**): Burst forward, reducing the distance between you and the aggressor, so that the stick ceases to be effective and is no longer dangerous. The assailant's forearm, or the stick itself, **slides** on the defender's forearm in continuation of its initial line of

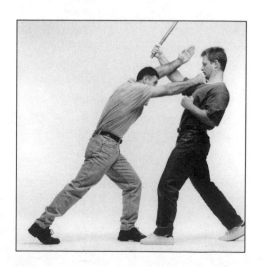

movement (with minimal change of direction). However, the attack must then be redirected away from the defender to form a complete defense. As a result of this kind of sliding defense, the impact with the defending forearm is minimal. When executing this defense, your head should be lowered and protected between your shoulders so that it avoids the line of danger.

4. *Threat from Behind at Close Range* (Chap. 4: **Neutralizing a Threat at Gunpoint**): Using **one arm**, with a sideways movement, you easily **deflect** the gun or the hand holding it. This action is performed simultaneously with a **body turn,** removing yourself from the line of fire and rapidly **advancing** towards the aggressor. One of the purposes of the advance is to bring you behind the gun and as far away from the line of fire as possible. Grabbing the forearm of the hand holding the gun will serve to keep it in place, preventing further use of the gun.

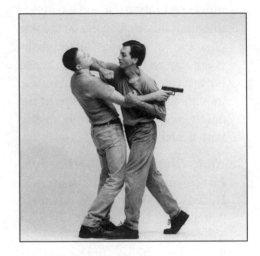

Chapter 12

Dealing with a Violent Incident:

Evaluation, Reaction, and Training Concepts

Handling the Incident

In this section we will summarize, with the aid of a general diagram, what happens to the human mind and body from the instant one perceives that an incident is occurring, until one takes positive action to deal with the situation.

A complete chain of stages and reactions ensues from the moment you perceive, through one of your senses, that something has occurred that is liable to endanger your own well-being or that of other people nearby. First, you must be conscious of the general nature of the danger you face as a result of the incident. You can then define the danger correctly, choose one of several possible courses of action, implement the course of action selected, and finally, proceed according to the new situation created as a result of the initiative you took.

On the next page, you will find a basic flow chart of the stages of human reaction to an incident such as being attacked:

Detailed explanation of the stages appearing in the diagram:

1. **Discernment of the occurrence** via the senses: sometimes you see the attack, e.g., a punch or kick, sometimes you may hear a noise or a cry of warning, and sometimes you feel someone grabbing your body, clothing, etc.

2. **Transfer of data to the brain**, by the nerves in the peripheral system: your eye perceives something and sends the information to your brain, your skin feels contact and conveys what is felt to the centers of sensation, etc.

3a. A process ensues, consisting mainly of **screening and identifying the above transmissions** from your sensory organs. Based on your past experience and knowledge, your brain "comprehends" the occurrences, translates them as danger, and issues a warning accordingly.

3b. As a result of the above, **a decision is made** in response to your understanding of the stimulus. Both in stages 3a and 3b, a number of functional areas of the brain participate in this decision-making process.

195

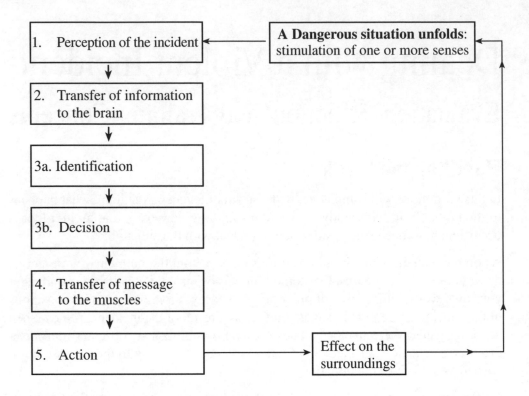

4. In order to **coordinate the reaction**, an appropriate message is conveyed by an electrochemical signal from the brain, via the nervous system, to the various muscle groups.

5. **Your muscles contract** with the proper timing and synchronization, in order to perform the action as decided and ordered by the brain.

The third stage (3a and 3b), which occurs in the brain, is the most complex and the most "problematic" part of the process. In the diagram this stage is divided into only two parts, but in reality, the brain process involves a vast number of stages, some of which occur in sequence and some simultaneously. Of all the stages, this is the one that is most subject to improvement and change, while the others, mostly a result of personal and hereditary traits, are very difficult to significantly improve!

Through learning processes and carefully designed training methods, accompanied by suitable practice, we can improve our technical and mental ability to identify incidents of a violent, dangerous nature, and function successfully in these situations by reducing our reaction time. In fact, the ultimate goal is to utilize these training methods not only to shorten our reaction time, but to enhance our ability to make **the correct decisions and perform the correct techniques at the correct time**.

Reaction time is really a measure of the interval between an unanticipated stimulus (such as a punch or a kick) and the beginning of the response to it. Reaction time reflects the brain's information-processing speed and the speed at which signals travel in the person's body. We can employ training methods to improve our ability to **recognize the stimulus** (attacks), **decide how to respond**, and learn to prepare the body to **initiate the correct physical response** without hesitation.

State Evaluation

If the attack takes you **completely by surprise**, you will act reflexively and intuitively. You will quickly draw upon reactions and behaviors acquired during your Krav Maga training and over the course of your life. Since decisions of this type are usually made on the **subconscious level**, it is more difficult for you to direct your actions and control them (consciously) in real time. Therefore, a considerable part of your training should be devoted to **internalizing patterns of movements and behavior**, to enable you to cope reflexively, intuitively, and without hesitation to surprise attacks.

On the other hand, when you are not taken by surprise and have enough time to consider your moves and decide consciously how to maneuver between one course of action and another, it is advisable to take one of the following measures, presented here in descending order of preference:

- **Seek a way to avoid entering the danger zone**. If possible, in most cases it is preferable simply not to enter into a confrontation, not to move close to the expected danger zone where a violent encounter may ensue.

- **Flee the scene**. If you are already involved in a violent confrontation, seek a way to execute a planned and controlled withdrawal from the scene **before you sustain real damage**. As wisely suggested in the Old Testament (the Book of Proverbs): *"...and before the quarrel flares up, abandon it."* While retreating, consider your moves carefully so as to avoid injury.

    Even in the midst of a fight, if you are truly in danger, it is advisable to flee the scene as quickly as possible, **if this can be done safely**. One's ego or desire to play the role of a hero should not be allowed to overpower one's instinct of self-preservation and natural intelligence. There is no shame at all in retreating if after considering all pertinent factors, it is tactically the best option.

    Note: You must also consider the fact that sometimes the harm done during your withdrawal or immediately afterwards is liable to be even **worse than the fight itself** (such as falling from a high place, injury from a passing car, leaving a third party who will be attacked more severely because of your absence, etc.), and act accordingly!

- **Using everyday objects found nearby**: If you cannot or do not wish to abandon the confrontation, try to find and use a nearby object or an item that you may be carrying on your person as an improvised weapon (as discussed in Chap. 7: **Using Everyday Objects as Defensive Weapons**).

- **Using your body as a weapon**: If you cannot find any object that might improve your chances, or do not have enough time to find such an item, then you must use "only" your body (and of course, your head!) for defense and attack. This is the main purpose of Krav Maga, and most of the techniques learned here belong to this category.

Physical and Mental Reactions Under Stress

In a state of **high situational anxiety**, you are naturally liable to be overwhelmed by fear, anger, and a host of other destructive feelings that will directly affect, and could significantly hinder the processes that occur in the brain during stages 3a and 3b (as previously described).

Given a high state of anxiety, your attention becomes **focused inward**, and your mental and physical actions therefore become deficient: your muscles contract unnecessarily, your perception of the surroundings becomes faulty, your decision-making process is prolonged, and the decisions you make are mostly erroneous and improperly implemented. Therefore, the purpose of the training methods presented here is to teach you how to deal more effectively with such negative feelings and the possible effect that they could have on you.

When you feel that you are in danger, a myriad of emotions is liable to enter your consciousness, and possibly overpower you, even without your awareness. The autonomous nervous system (that which is not subject to voluntary control) releases various substances into the bloodstream (such as adrenaline), which cause you to function at a different level than you are normally accustomed. We need training in order to **recognize this phenomenon** and the effect it has on our behavior in such extreme situations, and **learn to control it**. If we train under realistic conditions, our minds and bodies will become accustomed to the stress and will learn to function effectively even in such a state.

When in distress caused by physical threat, one will usually react in one of the following ways (the 3 F's): **Flight**: fleeing the scene of danger.

Freeze: a total paralysis of the motion system (or a drastic slowing down of that system). The person remains standing like a statue, with muscles unable to move any part of his (or her) body.

Fight: executing active combat moves, defense and attack, until the goal is ultimately achieved, i.e., the adversary cannot proceed with his hostile activity.

It is important to practice for each of the following possibilities and to develop the skill and ability to correctly function within each scenario: (1) To spot potential danger in advance and show restraint so as to avoid the confrontation. (2) If you are already involved in a violent confrontation, find the best and most effective way to flee the scene in a controlled and calculated manner, **without increasing the risk of injury to yourself**. (3) If you are fighting for your life (or the life of a third party), utilize the skills gained through your training with the defense and attack techniques needed for dealing with any possible violent threat. (4) If at any stage you feel a **state of paralysis** caused by fear or stress, learn ways to break that paralysis or state of inaction, so that you can act according to all the feasible options open to you. This is achieved through training and practice.

Training Methods Used to Improve Ability

Having explained the nature of the processes occurring in your mind and body, we will now discuss training methods geared towards achieving a general improvement in the ability to act quickly and correctly when the need arises. In some methods we will focus on the **identification** system only, in others we will concentrate on the **decision-making** system, and in certain methods of training we will deal with other specific segments of the process or with the entire process itself.

Based on the theory presented in the flow chart at the beginning of this chapter, the following is the basic structure of the different training methods. First, we will present the methods devised for improving the observation, recognition, and identification of the action or the attack movement that an adversary is liable to perform. To do this, we must implement the following stages in the flow chart:

a. First range of methods   b. Second range of methods

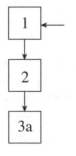

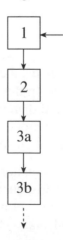

Using the **first range of methods**, you will stand in place and observe the various attacks that are directed against you. In this way you will learn to recognize possible patterns and sequences of movements, and later to train your mind and body in the steps that must be taken against them. With the **second range of methods**, you will think and become aware of the actions and defense(s) that you must execute, and the decisions you must make, in order to foil the aggressor's actions. When practicing these training methods, it is important that you remain calm while observing your partner's attacks, without the need to take any actions or fulfill any standards. (See the following section: **Observation – Watching a Series of Attacks**.)

When we remove the first and second stages from the main flow chart, we obtain a special range of training drills, which will be discussed in depth in the next chapter: **Additional Training Methods; How to Use this Book**. We refer here to **mental training**, in which the main component is **imagination**. In these techniques, the student acts alone, either with his brain only or with the inclusion of physical movements as well. Different combinations of these stages will represent the various methods as follows:

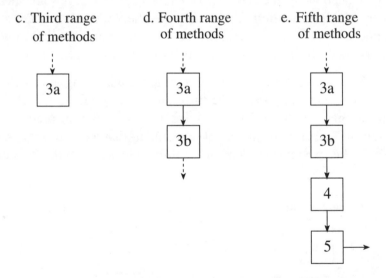

c. Third range
of methods

d. Fourth range
of methods

e. Fifth range
of methods

In these training methods, the stimulus is supplied by **the images that you create in your imagination**. In the third range of methods (c), your brain will practice "seeing" an action and then perform some sort of identification procedure. In the fourth (d), you will go through the identification process, decide what action to take, and perform in your imagination the necessary moves, defenses, attacks, etc.

The appropriate counteraction that you have chosen can be performed either in the air or with training aids, such as a sack, dummy, etc. A more advanced training activity in the fifth range of methods (e) might be, for example, to imagine a fight against several assailants.

In the illustration, the second, third, fourth, and fifth ranges of methods are marked with dotted arrows. They are dotted to show that when you imagine the physical action, you are likely to involve the perceiving senses, the peripheral nervous system, and the muscles but only to a minimal degree. In the fifth range, you can perform the action in space without affecting your surroundings, or on a target, thus affecting your surroundings. This stage is therefore marked by a solid arrow.

There is a wide variety of training methods, encompassing all the stages (1 through 5) listed in the main flow chart. Some are based on **perception via the senses**: sight, hearing, touch, or other sensation, while others are intended to drill you in **quick decision-making**, rapid or precise movements, and even functioning under more stressful condition.

Observation – Watching a Series of Attacks

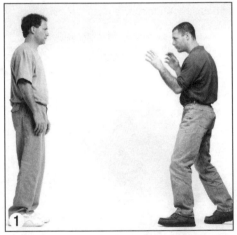

This activity begins, for example, with the observer in a passive stance. The attacker starts from a general outlet stance or any other position.

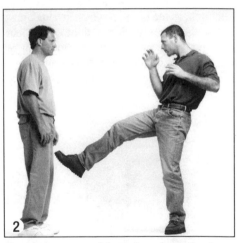

Commencement of the series of attacks: long-range attack, such as a regular kick to the groin.

This is an example of the basic training method, which involves recognition of movement and of how the assailant's possible attacks are created. The observer watches a series of attacks and internalizes the courses that their movements follow. Since you, as the observer, do not have to execute defenses, you can remain calm, greatly facilitating your absorption of the attacker's movements. This is the first stage in developing the defender's ability to identify an attack and take effective action against it.

The assailant appears also in the training and practicing phase. You, **as the attacker**, utilize techniques, applying them in different variations and combinations, while passing through different ranges and delivering accurate attacks to vulnerable points.

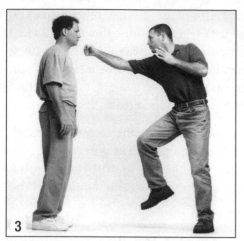

Continuation at medium range, as the attacker moves in with a straight punch to your chin. Although, as the observer, you can sometimes look at the attacking limb and the course that it follows, most of the time you should not be focusing your attention or looking at any single attack, but rather should be constantly observing the entire picture.

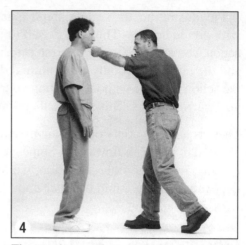

The attacker continues to burst forward; the range between you is decreased further as he delivers a roundhouse punch.

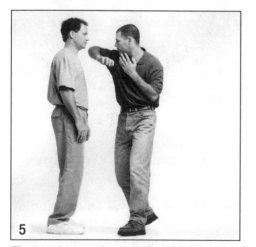

The attacker continues to decrease the range, e.g., by moving diagonally forward, and delivers a horizontal elbow strike.

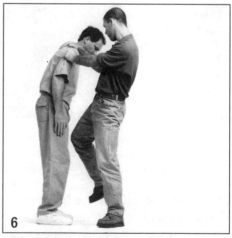

The attacker concludes this series of attacks by sending a knee kick to your groin.

In the role of the attacker, you can strike lightly at vulnerable points **if protective equipment is used**. From the attacker's standpoint, the onset of movement represents the moment that you recognize the fact that you are actually going to attack. This exercise requires a minimal level of aggression. Those engaged in Krav Maga training use this basic drill in order to acquire and maintain the ability to deliver the proper attack, at the proper time, from the appropriate distance and angle, thus enhancing their ability to perform in the fight. Training should include an attacker starting from a variety of positions and angles relative to the one who is observing him.

Change of Action during the Initial Response

The perception of a particular stimulus initiated the chain of actions defined in stages 1 through 5, and you, the person involved in the incident, reacted and behaved in one way or another. Now, consider the possibility that **another stimulus**, in addition to the first, has also reached the brain. A change of action will be possible only if your attention remains "open" to new perceptions, and can process the new stimulus while performing the action triggered by the first.

Another condition for changing an action during an incident, is that process number 5 has not yet reached its final stages, because then it is more difficult, though still possible to a certain degree, to stop or alter the initial action. Therefore, if you **keep your attention and senses open** to perceive a new sensation and do not concentrate only on the original action, the greater the possibility (and ease) of changing your action during the entire incident.

Neutralizing the Danger in All Its Aspects

When an attack takes place, or when a threat exists, you must **perform all actions necessary to neutralize any and all possibilities of getting hurt**! This general principle means that all aspects of the danger must be dealt with in the order of priority as dictated by the series of actions and the structure of the movements, and according to your timing and instant readiness, as detailed below:

a. **First stage**: Preventing the attack from reaching its target, i.e., the punch does not hit the chin, the choke hold does not block the carotid artery or the trachea, the bullet misses the intended target, the swing of the stick is deflected, causing it to miss your head, a stab is stopped before the knife reaches your body, etc.

b. **Second stage**: Preventing the immediate possibility of the aggressor delivering another, similar attack (especially with a weapon) or a different attack, by "dealing with" the assailant. In cases of **threats or attacks with a weapon**, you sometimes have to gain control of the weapon and at the same time, or as soon as possible, neutralize the assailant. Now it is the time to ascertain the presence (or absence) of **other assailants** that so far you have failed to notice.

c. **Third stage**: Conclusion of the action, i.e., creating a situation in which the attacker cannot (or does not wish to) pursue the attack further. If a weapon is involved, conclusion of the action will generally include **disarming the assailant**.

The ranking of priorities when dealing with multiple attacks or attackers is specifically described in Chap. 10: **Defense against Two Armed Assailants**.

If it is possible and you choose to **flee the scene quickly**, foiling the attempted attack, the incident will end as early as the first stage. A controlled withdrawal can also be executed **after a defensive action**, e.g., blocking the assailant's stabbing hand after delivering one or two decisive counterattacks.

Generally, we strive to **include a counterattack against the aggressor** as part of the first step. At other times, this action will be preceded by measures meant to prevent the attacker from making further use of his body or weapon. When a **weapon** is involved, the second stage will include two parts: dealing with the assailant and limiting his ability to use the weapon. This will depend on the type of weapon and the nature of the attack.

Note: The different stages of neutralizing the danger are sometimes executed simultaneously.

Following are two examples from Chap. 1: **Defense against Knife Attack**. Using these examples, we will analyze the self-defense techniques used and examine the guiding principles of neutralizing the various components of the danger.

1. **Forearm defense against downward knife stab – regular hold, and counterattack**: In this case, the defense is integrated with a counterattack, executed either simultaneously with the defense or immediately afterwards. The first stage is to stop the attack. The second stage (integrated with the first) is the counterattack. As early as possible, we add a hand control, geared towards restricting the movement of the stabbing hand in order to minimize the danger of the assailant using his knife again. The third stage is to bring the incident to an end, through additional counterattacks, and by disarming the adversary, as necessary and according to the situation.

2. **Techniques based on attacks** that precede the adversary in anticipation of his actions, also include the same stages, even though they are not always clearly defined. For example: *Stab, Regular Hold – Kick to the Groin* or *Stab, Oriental Hold – Kick to the Chin*. In both techniques, you execute a fast, powerful attack that hurts and stops the assailant before he is within range to use the knife effectively. In these techniques, we encounter the first two stages: preventing the attack from landing and attacking the assailant, combining both in a single movement. The final stage of the incident will depend on the result of this

Chapter 13

Additional Training Methods; How to Use this Book

Underlying Principles in Krav Maga Training

In the introductory chapter **What is Krav Maga?** we set forth the general principles upon which the system is based. In this chapter, we will detail specific principles pertaining to training and practice in order to achieve the greatest possible results as a self-defense practitioner and competent street fighter.

Action from a Position of Disadvantage

In Krav Maga, the various self-defense techniques are applied when your position is **inferior** relative to that of the assailant. For example, in freeing oneself from a hold, the defender must begin the defense from a position in which he (or she) is being held strongly, a situation that greatly restricts and endangers the defender. If you are defending yourself against a specific attack, it must be assumed that the attack has started and is already being applied against you, posing a most serious threat to your safety and survival.

In reality, you may be able to react earlier if you observe the attack from its inception or if you are ready and anticipate it in advance. Since this is not always the case, we address in this book techniques that are needed for neutralizing both the attack and the attacker when the defender responds from various states of readiness.

The defense technique must be **effective, motion-efficient, and fast**. Therefore, as soon as you implement the defensive move, you will respond as early as possible with the counterattack(s) or rapidly leave the scene. Remember that while a defense may be performed successfully against a specific attack (freeing you from immediate danger), the defense itself in most cases does not completely eliminate the threat to one's safety.

Therefore, we place considerable emphasis in Krav Maga on applying a **highly effective and aggressive counterattack** (or a minor one when required), or a **controlled retreat** from the scene of the incident. These actions are to be taken simultaneously with the initial defense or immediately afterwards. This combination of defense and counterattack helps to **eliminate the threat in its entirety**. The concept of delivering the counterattack simultaneously with the defense is an essential element of most Krav Maga techniques.

Another principle associated with many Krav Maga techniques is to **prevent the assailant from taking further action with his weapon**, hampering his ability to use it again or move freely with it. We also strive to restrict the moves of an **unarmed assailant**, stopping him from delivering additional punches, kicks, etc., or from locating an object that he could use as a weapon against us.

Training with a Partner

Krav Maga training includes the following methods: Practicing punches and kicks on a punching bag and to other targets, such as focus mitts; performing techniques as "dry-drills" (i.e., without a partner); mental training to further develop the proper mental state and physical skills, etc. Fundamentally, the main elements in training focus upon **using a partner to offer resistance**, and to create an opposition that enhances a sense of reality.

At the outset, it is suggested that practice drills with a partner be **relatively slow**. This will allow the participants to better understand and internalize the exercises, the techniques, the underlying principles of the system, and the different elements that exist within the confrontation.

Practice should **simulate a real incident**. However, participants must try to refrain from striking one another with maximum force. Obviously, they should not leave the training session bruised and battered to the point of being unable to continue their regular routine... or even worse, being unable to respond to an attack in the "real world" as a result of their injuries.

Note: Careless training has extremely negative effects on the morale and the mental attitude, both of which are essential during a real-life confrontation. In addition, **careless training may cause irreversible health-related damage**! Therefore, anyone who trains in Krav Maga should carefully review the relevant material contained in Chapter 14: **Safety in Training**, and implement the suggestions found therein.

Practice with Variations

When we are concerned with defense and release techniques, and with counterattacks, training should begin with the practice of definite techniques. This is called a "closed" or "defined" skill. Once the student has partially internalized the basic defenses and the principles behind them, he (or she) may proceed to practice at a more advanced level, by having to defend against slight to moderate variations in the basic attack.

Training sessions are conducted as though you are standing inside a sphere, so that attacks can come from any direction, at any height and from various positions. This is called "open-skill" training. Thus, for example, you will apply a defined defensive technique against a specific attack while executing the correct defense and the corresponding counterattack. Then you will execute defenses against the same or similar attack, coming from different angles and being delivered at different heights. You will eventually practice defenses against the same or similar attack, but this time in a state of motion or while your movements are restricted, e.g., by standing against a wall or behind a desk, performing the defenses while sitting down, then while lying down, and so forth. All of the above defenses are executed against specific attacks coming from different angles, speeds, and rhythms, taking care that each defense will follow through with a counterattack delivered as early as possible.

Since no two people act in exactly the same way (and even the same person may act differently while in a similar situation!), it is advisable to **train with different partners**, varying in height, weight, agility, etc., rather than become accustomed to one partner only. The concluding stage in this type of training is to defend yourself against **two or more attackers**.

From Technique to Principle, and Back to Technique
The principles outlined in this book embrace a wide variety of techniques: some are precisely defined, while others are not. As soon as you are able to recognize the general principles supporting a specific technique, you will improve your perception of those underlying principles as well as become aware of other techniques that are based on the same or similar principles.

In performing one technical exercise, bear in mind the principles behind it. Therefore, you actually improve your ability to perform several techniques. This contributes towards improving your "open skill" response in related subjects. This is of crucial importance, because it **develops your ability to perform successfully when facing variations in the attack**, which will call for proper adjustment of the specific technique that you were practicing. The ability to defend against these variations of the "basic" attack simulates true-life situations, which are always somewhat different from those conditions that exist in a controlled training session.

This is the true benefit inherent in an integrated and fully comprehensive training system: the ability to regulate your decision-making process, to practice solving new problems as well as understanding how to deal with variations of known problems.

Basics of Training

First of all you should read this book carefully from beginning to end, and make sure that you thoroughly understand all of the system's central concepts. Once again, we stress that you must read Chapter 14: **Safety in Training** with extra care **before beginning** any physical training whatsoever! Of course, one should train only under the direct supervision of a highly qualified, duly certified Krav Maga instructor.

It is also very important to make sure that you **thoroughly understand** all of the technical explanations corresponding to each photograph, each exercise, and each chapter. We recommend that you carefully study the various techniques presented (along with their underlying principles) and search for the similarities between them. It is these similarities and principles that turn the collection of exercises into a consolidated, logical, and useful system that can be employed against real-life dangers that you may encounter.

Some chapters also include explanations and suggestions on how to act with proper tactics in various problematic scenarios. This goes a step beyond dealing with a variety of specific attacks. The greatness of the masterfighter lies in his ability to use the minimum possible physical action and strength in order to win a confrontation. At times, it is also possible to **defeat one's adversary mentally**, with no physical contact whatsoever; the opponent succumbs before the fight even begins!

Once you have read this book and gained a general picture of the myriad of dangers you are liable to encounter, it is time to practice a specific defensive technique against a **specific type of assault or threat**, e.g., an assailant armed with a stick, knife, or handgun. It is advisable to begin your practice in the order that the techniques appear in this book, although it is also possible to train in any other logical order that is appropriate for you.

Practicing Alone
Following are some important points to remember when training alone: Begin your session with a **light warm-up** to stimulate blood circulation, stretch your muscles, and enhance the flexibility and range of movement in your joints. It is essential to avoid placing too much strain on body systems that are not ready for such activity, since this may cause immediate or delayed damage! As always, before engaging in any kind of physical activity, **you should first consult your personal physician and obtain medical clearance!**

After selecting a specific technique and using the book to study it thoroughly, stand and **imagine an assailant** executing the same attack, consistent with the one shown in the photographs. Begin from the same outlet stance pictured, and then slowly execute the moves demonstrated by the defender in the photographs. You can also **use a mirror**, to check whether your movements and positions match those of the defender in the photographs.

A basic, defensive technique can usually be executed in a **single** movement. However, if the technique is more complicated, you should divide it into a **series** of movements. Divide the exercises according to the photographs and the corresponding explanations. If necessary, you can train separately on each stage and then combine the stages together in order to form the entire technique. You can also benefit from a partner who is watching you and helping to correct any mistakes in your movements.

Practicing with a Partner

Once you understand and can conceptualize the technique, and have practiced it in the air against an imaginary assailant, you are ready to begin training with a partner. Both you and your partner should execute the attack, the defense, and the counter-attack as shown in the photographs. Act slowly. Your partner will carefully perform the attack "with the intention to injure" you. At first, you will slowly and calmly execute the techniques you have practiced as if performing them in "slow motion."

Remember: Your body should be ready for the physical contact between you and your partner.

In order to effectively increase the power and speed of both the attack and the defense, especially against a partner attacking with a weapon, it is advisable that the "assailant" use **padded forearm guards**. Only after taking the required safety measures and achieving the initial skill through slow, calculated practice, should you start practicing defenses against stronger, faster attacks.

In addition to training with a partner, you should also re-read relevant parts of this book in order to find additional points related to the techniques you are practicing.

Training Methods for Defense against Sharp-Edged Weapons and Blunt Objects

Once you have practiced the various techniques and feel comfortable applying them, you can proceed to a more advanced level of training. By using advanced training methods and didactic games, you can improve your ability to quickly identify a specific attack, immediately deciding how to respond with a suitable defense and simultaneous counterattack. For example:

Different Situations: Your partner, in the role of the assailant, will change his position from one attack to another. The assailant will attack from a **variety of distances** (ranges) and angles, and employ **different types of attacks**, while armed with a knife or a stick.

Late Perception: Your partner will hide his weapon behind his back, and then abruptly start his attack. You, the defender, will stand in place, look straight ahead, and allow him to attack you from different positions and directions, leaving you with less time to recognize the attack and react. This method will improve your alertness and ability to respond in **short-notice, real-life situations** and allow you to achieve the desired result. This occurs by responding to the attack, without knowing in advance the nature of the specific attack being directed at you.

Note: In real-life situations, under no circumstances should you permit a potential assailant to place himself in a position so close that your safety may be endangered!

Multiple Attacks: In this case the assailant will not execute a **single attack**, but rather a **series of attacks** (identical or different). Your defenses and counterattacks must neutralize both of the dangers posed to you, i.e., the specific threat(s) of the attacks and of the attacker himself.

Again, we stress that a **planned retreat** at the proper time and in the correct direction is sometimes the best course of action! Alternatively, you can increase your "safety distance" from the attacker, and position yourself so that you are ready to perform the appropriate defensive techniques and counterattacks.

Eyes Closed: While standing with your eyes closed, your partner assumes the stance of an assailant in the midst of an attack with his weapon held about 16"-20" (40-50 cm) from your body. Your partner must "alert" you by giving you some sort of signal. As soon as you open your eyes in response to the prearranged signal, quickly identify the danger and perform a suitable technique against the specific attack offered by your partner. This is the basic stage of training with your eyes closed.

Additional Training Methods – Threat with a Firearm

Once you have practiced the basic techniques against various threats with a handgun, rifle or submachine gun, feel that you are able to defend against the basic threats, and understand the principles behind the gun defenses, you may then continue your training by creating more "dangerous" scenarios. Such training will improve your speed in **recognizing the attack** and making **tactical decisions** on how to respond appropriately. These additional scenarios will expand the range of situations in which you will be prepared to successfully respond. You can also apply some of the training methods described earlier for defending against sharp or blunt objects and threats with a firearm.

Note: The words "**gun**" and "**firearm**" as used here, are generic terms for handgun, submachine gun, and rifle.

Advanced Training Methods
Practicing Neutralization of a Threat Accompanied by Grabbing or Shoving: The assailant grabs you and also pushes and leads you, while threatening you with his gun. This requires performing the necessary technique with your movement being restricted, or having to defend while walking or being pushed.

Practicing Neutralization in Different Directions: This simulates a situation where an innocent **third party** is present on your right or your left side, and might be in the line of fire once you have deflected the gun in his or her direction. In this situation, you must apply a technique that positively ensures deflection of the firearm in a **direction that does not endanger** the person next to you.

Practicing Neutralization of a Threat in a Seated Position: It is important to practice gun defenses while sitting in a chair with the assailant relatively close to you. It is also possible to perform similar exercises while seated in a motor vehicle. This is particularly relevant due to the large and ever-increasing number of "motorized crimes" worldwide, such as car-jacking and other attacks directed at drivers or passengers, from both outside and inside the vehicle.

Playing the Role: The better and more realistic your partner plays his (or her) role as the "assailant" while giving orders, acting nervously or erratically and even "insulting" you, moving, shoving, grabbing, etc., the better you will function under the stress of a genuine confrontation.

Integration and Combination

Integration and Combination of Situations, Techniques, and Training Methods: Playing the part of the assailant is crucial to the development of a "street fighter." This is especially true when the defender knows as little as possible in advance about the impending threat or attack. Role playing should involve a wide variety of attacks and defensive options as specified in the following examples:

Defending from a **seated position** against a **stick attack**. Sometimes you will use the chair for defense and attack, and sometimes "only" your body.

Consider practicing the defense against **knife stab**, when the attacker is **holding you by your clothes** with his free hand while executing the same stab **several times** in rapid succession. In your defense, you will have to deal with the repeated attacks and execute counterattacks as quickly as possible.

It is extremely challenging to practice the defense techniques while initially having your **eyes closed**, and then suddenly opening them in response to an audible signal, a slight punch, or a grab from the assailant. You must instantly recognize the threat and immediately execute the appropriate defensive technique, as effectively and accurately as possible.

In addition, you, as the defender, should move around, and the attacker should emerge from behind a shelter or barrier in such a way that you will identify the attack only **at the last possible moment**. Just as you discern the attacking partner, you must identify his actions and defend, counterattack, or increase distance, according to the incident and the specific type of attack. In order to broaden the variety of possible scenarios and incidents, create **combinations of different training challenges** from the selections given below.

The following represents most of the factors that can be combined in order to create a training scenario:

- One type of attack combined with another type of attack.
- The defender performing from a fighting stance or a neutral stance.
- Changes in the angle of attack; altering the assailant's position during the attack.
- Changing the site (environment) where the actual training takes place as well as the time of day, interchanging a variety of weapons used by the assailant.
- It is also important to employ different numbers of assailants participating in the training session, all acting against the defender at the same time, from various angles, posing different or identical threats.

There are additional training techniques as well, but those noted above are more than enough for extended training. You should remember that the name of the game is **practice and more practice**, but do it creatively and in an intelligent, challenging way so that true development and growth is fostered.

Mental Training

We are faced with the problem of how to train a person to deal with life-and-death situations. Obviously, the participants cannot be killed or seriously harmed and then somehow returned to their previous uninjured condition in order to repeat the exercise and correct any mistakes. The real challenge is to put the trainee into a **realistic, true-to-life training format** that raises problems and causes stress, but without threatening his (or her) life or well-being as could occur in a real situation.

Why must we simulate a real-life violent confrontation? Is technical study not sufficient in itself, without the need for special mental training? The answer is negative! Mental training is crucial to one's ability to survive a violent confrontation. At the moment when your life is in jeopardy, you must deal not only with the source of the danger (the attacker), but also with your own mind and body responses to the life-threatening situation. In fact, a **unified relationship exists between mind and body** that deals with the fear and stress experienced during a violent confrontation. How one deals with fear and mental stress will directly impact one's ability to make the correct decisions in time and at the required speed, as well as the physical performance of the suitable techniques that have been committed to memory through previous training.

Dealing with a violent confrontation usually creates mental stress and often triggers intense destructive feelings and emotions such as fear, anxiety, hate, rage, etc. Engaging in mental training will solve these problems by improving one's self-control, allowing better control over one's emotions and rendering the process of decision-making faster and more accurate. The autonomous nervous system causes the secretion of large quantities of adrenaline into the blood. In this state, the person may either **freeze, run away**, or **fight**.

It is clear that freezing on the spot (although it may sometimes serve certain animals as a defense against predators) is ineffective in most situations that we are liable to encounter. If the response is either to run or to fight, this choice must be made in a **well-controlled manner**, with our senses open to absorb relevant stimuli and information from the surroundings, which is done much better when our attention is not limited by feelings and emotions. "Freezing" must be deleted, therefore, from our instinctive range of reactions. If the person ceases to move, he must do so out of some tactical decision, and **not because he has lost control** over his actions.

It has been documented that there are athletes who achieve much better results in training than in actual competition. This happens because, during competition, the mental strain and pressure of the situation often "rob" them of a large portion of their physical and mental resources. They are not exclusively concentrating on the actions required of them, and are therefore losing the energy needed to achieve their best results. Psychologists and special coaches help such athletes to better control the stress and instill a feeling of confidence in them.

People in all walks of life, from performers that appear before tens of thousands of people to stockbrokers that control fortunes of tens of millions of dollars, sometimes find it difficult to withstand the heavy mental pressure under which they must function. Some even turn to drugs, thus bringing themselves closer to self-destruction.

Clearly, it is our **inner mental resources** that enable us to function effectively and properly in our everyday life. We should be able in each experience to cope successfully with our subjective emotions and feelings, and to come out of every incident while retaining the upper hand. We must also learn from the very fact of the confrontation. Thus, the incident helps us to understand the forces acting upon us, and strengthens our mental and spiritual capabilities.

Ultimately, solving the problem presented at the beginning of this section: training for life or death situations **without getting hurt**, will be achieved only with the **integration of mental training into the overall training regimen**. This is the way to develop and fine-tune the required mental powers. It is necessary to practice and use this mental training in combination with physical, technical, and tactical training.

It is known that the human body reacts to images created in the imagination and in the subconscious in the same or similar manner as it reacts to images and sensations absorbed from the outside. We will use this fact to enhance our ability to deal with danger. There is no fundamental difference in our reaction, given an image that appears as the result of **external stimulation** or out of our **internal creation**. The close relationship existing between the imagined picture and the imaginer's mental state and his subconscious explain the reason behind mental training. Simply, the **subconscious**, which is the source of feelings that hinder a person's mental and physical capabilities during a confrontation, is exercised while the person "views" or "pictures" the imagined incident.

Using this approach, you, the trainee, act with your imagination only, and at a time when you are relatively relaxed and comfortable. For instance, while sitting in a train, a bus, or an airplane or while waiting for your dentist, taking advantage of your free time. Imagine a scene in which you are in a certain place, and a violent assailant tries to attack you. Try to visualize the assailant, note his (or her) dress, observe the attack techniques used by the assailant, and what weapon he (or she) is holding. Also note your own mental state and position at that moment.

By picturing the threat and imagining the proper tactics and defensive techniques, your nerves and muscles are much more likely to respond to a real-life danger without succumbing to stress interference. Mental training allows techniques and tactics to become second nature to you. It "imprints" upon you the techniques and tactics that you have learned, so that under the stress of an attack, **your physical response is made without conscious thought or hesitation**. Mental training will also familiarize you with just how a life-threatening situation unfolds, how it looks and feels, thereby defusing the impact of the stress and shock phenomena when you are actually faced with such a threat in real life.

There are two alternative methods for observing an incident: (1) As though you were **watching a movie screen**, in which the figures (including yourself) are performing before you. (2) Viewing it as though you were an **active participant**, functioning within the incident. The second approach should be emphasized, as it better simulates the point of view a defender usually has during a violent confrontation.

The Technique

Imagine the incident in the different stages, according to the various possibilities for its conclusion. First, allow your imagined assailant to succeed in his attack, and see yourself "injured." "Feel" the attack injuring you and causing you pain, as if you are the "loser" in the incident. Imagine the incident again and again, in slow motion, **each time improving your position and performance**. When you imagine the incident, apply more and more effective defenses, and execute counterattacks that become gradually stronger and faster. In the end, visualize yourself as the winner, repeatedly overcoming the assailant with effective defenses and counterattacks.

Most of the focus should be on **visualizing yourself as the "winner"** in order to engrave this outcome in your mind, to increase the chances that this will also occur in a **real-life fight** for your survival. The very fact that you are aware of the possibility that you may "lose" or get hurt, will lessen your fear of actually getting hurt, and significantly **improve your ability to function under pressure**. Once you have reached the stage that you have defeated the aggressor in your imagination, you can proceed to imaginary practice of another attack technique, in another situation, against another assailant.

In the advanced stages of mental training, you should imagine the **entire fight**, an extended confrontation, against an assailant. You can combine imagination with actual physical actions, that is, you imagine the attacks, actions, and behavior of the imaginary assailant(s), while you physically perform the necessary defenses and counterattacks, initiate attacks, and change tactics. During this activity you should be "conscious" of the "person" before you, and strive to "see" his (or her) responses to your actions and the effect that they have on your adversary. Practice these actions **slowly, and with close attention to detail**. The importance of the imaginary fight or combat lies in the creation of successive, moving images and scenarios.

In addition, it is clear that it also works the other way around, i.e., all the "regular" physical practice of defensive techniques and tactics, as well as hand-to-hand combat, also trains, improves your readiness, and prepares you for the mental confrontation; the reason being that when we train physically, our mind is being exercised too, therefore the more stressful the training, mentally and physically, the better.

Finally, it should be noted that despite the importance of mental training, in the end it is your body that will ultimately perform the physical actions that will save your life or the lives of those nearby. Therefore, it is no less important to **improve your physical fitness**, and particularly **your ability to absorb an attack and ignore the pain** that might be caused during the confrontation. As a result, you will increase your ability to confidently and successfully handle an assailant posing a genuine threat and, when needed, overcome him more easily and effectively without being hindered by hesitation or self-inflicted emotional and physical interference.

A Real-Life Story

Never underestimate your opponent: A former world chess champion is riding on a train in central Europe, and a man sitting next to him suggests a game of chess. He refuses, of course, as he sees no point in it: He personally knows all the world-class chess players and it is therefore clear that the difference in skill is much too great. The other man urges him on, and in the end he agrees to play just one game. The champion plays carelessly, and loses. The passenger asks for another game. As the chess champion knows that if he plays more seriously this time he will certainly win, he refuses. The other man keeps imploring him and he finally consents, but though he plays to the best of his ability, he loses again. Now it is the champion who demands another game, but despite all his efforts, and to his great surprise as he plays at his best, he loses for a third time. He asks the passenger: "Who are you, and where did you learn to play like that?" The man answers that he lives in one of the small villages in the area, has never been out of the country, and has always played only with his friends. To his great regret, he says, the train has now reached his stop and he must get off, and thanks for the enjoyable contest. He then disappears, leaving the world champion to wonder about this strange incident for the rest of his life...

Chapter 14

Safety in Training

Acquiring the skills necessary to cope with an assailant in a violent confrontation or an enemy in battle requires training. Training in a fighting method means dealing physically (from light to full contact) as well as mentally with one or more partners. Training also involves the utilizing of different types of professional equipment such as punching bag, focus mitts, and other training pads or contact suits, used to build one's skills. Techniques can also be improved and refined by performing them as "dry drills", i.e., without the interaction of a partner or the resistance of a punching bag, in essence, by physically performing them "to the air."

Our objective is for the student to participate in all types of training **without getting hurt**. For this we need a suitable place in which to train, an appropriate code of behavior, the proper equipment, and a gradual approach to enhance learning and experience intense training. Fulfilling these conditions will prevent the occurrence of most dangers and minimize the chances of injury. In this chapter, we will present guidelines for achieving this sound objective.

Undoubtedly, some conflict does exist when balancing between the following two contradictory approaches of critical importance: training methods and scenarios that place stress on the trainee and simulate street attacks under real-life conditions, as opposed to training methods free of factors that are liable to cause debilitating or serious injury to the participants. The Krav Maga discipline has always insisted on **combining these two opposite approaches**, and training its disciples in an almost real atmosphere, without inflicting any unnecessary bodily harm.

Physical Check-up

A physical check-up is a **must** for both student and instructor, in order to allay any fear of insufficient physical fitness. The student and instructor must be fit enough for the type of energetic activity and physical challenges usually found in Krav Maga. Nevertheless, even people with certain physical limitations (whether slight or even more serious) can train in Krav Maga, though **under special instruction with the necessary medical supervision**, and achieve impressive results. In Israel, special Krav Maga training courses were given to people suffering from severe handicaps, whether as a result of acts of war or from an early age. In many cases, the participants graduated with astonishing results despite their limitations!

Before engaging in any Krav Maga training, one should always obtain medical clearance. Physicians who are reviewing (judging) the appropriateness of such training for an individual, **should be made aware of the high level of physical contact and cardiovascular stress placed on the participant**. It must also be emphasized that a person learning from a handbook or a video must be especially · careful while practicing, whether he (or she) is training alone or with a partner, since **they lack the personal supervision and the tutelage of an "on-hand" experienced certified Krav Maga instructor**.

The Training Place

Any place where people can engage in sports and physical training, in our case, Krav Maga, is considered a **training place**. This can be an athletic club, a lawn, a beach, your living room, etc. The type and the place of training must be compatible.

Before practice begins, any object that is likely to cause injury to the participants **must be moved aside**. When training on a gym floor covered with mats, take great care to ensure that the mats are firmly attached to each other with no space in between and **with no possibility of slipping**. It is best if the entire mat-covered floor is then covered with a tightly stretched tarpaulin or plastic sheet with no folds, gaps, or tears.

The training place should be **well ventilated** to ensure an adequate supply of fresh air. An unlimited supply of drinking water must be on hand, and during hot weather participants must drink water **during the training session** itself.

Note: The entrance and the exit to the training place should permit the **convenient passage** of two people carrying a third, in case of injury.

A first aid kit must always be on hand. It should be well stocked and equipped with items suited to a wide range of injuries, from the very slight to the most serious. Be sure to inspect the kit and replenish it as required. The kit must be readily accessible and its location made known to everyone participating in the training session.

A Krav Maga student should regularly train in different places, including places **where he might actually be faced with violent confrontation**. If he does not do so, unfamiliar surroundings are liable to hinder his mental ability, and when this occurs, his physical capability suffers as well. Therefore, when arriving at a training site other than your regular one, be sure to carefully inspect the location for obvious or hidden safety risks. Of course, **a first aid kit must be brought** to the training site as well.

It goes without saying that a training studio must also meet the standard **local and state requirements** with regards to safety and sanitary conditions.

Dress and Appearance

Clothing and equipment must be appropriate for the training, and vice versa. Before the session begins, the student shall **remove any objects or jewelry**, that are liable to endanger himself (or herself) or others participating in the lesson. Such items include, for example, wrist watches, necklaces, rings, and earrings.

Note: Special precautions must be taken if a student (man or woman) wears glasses or has long hair, long fingernails, etc.

Training attire should be aesthetic and complete, without accessories liable to endanger the participants such as belt buckle, open zipper, torn clothing, dangling pockets, etc.

Safety equipment and **protective gear** should always be appropriate to the type of training. The degree of force on impact shall be adapted to the protective gear that the student is wearing, so as to **avoid excessive force** that may result in injury. Bandages, boxing wrap, and guards shall be complete, worn in a proper manner, and must have no pins or sharp edges.

Knowing all of the above, it is essential to train in **different types of clothing**: from swimsuit and light summer wear, to thick, heavy winter clothes. In order to prepare for real-life situations, the trainee must feel comfortable performing self-defense techniques and fighting drills in any kind of clothing, and should not become accustomed to training in one type only!

Warm-up

The purpose of warm-up is to prepare the student, physically and mentally, for training. The warm-up must suit the type of training to follow. Warm-up should be **gradual**, and include activation of the different body systems.

When faced with an actual, violent encounter, one obviously cannot ask the assailant for time to warm up... At every moment, and in a split second, one must be ready, physically and mentally, to take the proper action and handle the adversary without a warm-up. At times like this, the necessary aid comes from the autonomous nervous system, whose purpose is to deal with such events by injecting naturally stimulating substances such as adrenaline into the bloodstream. However, in sessions where one chooses to train without a warm-up, special care must be taken **to avoid sudden, overly strenuous activities** that might cause harm.

It is recommended that a light warm-up be performed before proceeding to the physical activity described in the various learning methods and techniques presented in this book. This light warm-up lasts from 10 to 15 minutes and usually includes

stretching exercises, to stimulate circulation, speed up the cardiovascular system, and increase flexibility in the muscles and joints, and also **light power exercises**, such as push-ups, sit-ups, and squats: deep knee bends. It is also recommended that the warm-up include some **fighting games** and exercise some **basic techniques** of Krav Maga.

Code of Behavior – Self-Discipline; Following the Instructions of the Instructor or Session Leader

When training with a partner (or partners), **without the presence of an instructor**, it is recommended to decide who will lead the session. This person will be called the "**session leader**."

The key to training safely and avoiding unnecessary injury, is **proper behavior**. This is based on self-discipline and on following the instructions of the session leader.

Caution: When training alone or with a partner according to written instructions, the absence of an experienced instructor makes it especially important to maintain a high standard of responsibility and strictly adhere to the safety rules.

The instructions must be followed in order to achieve **uniformity in group behavior**; a large group of students involved in a training session should always move in pre-arranged directions in order to reduce the chance of collision among participants.

When practicing a particular technique, the trainee is supposed to execute the various attacks and defenses when he (or she) is in a **"cool" emotional state**. One must not become angry with one's partner (or adversary) or act out of rage, anger or fear, and of course, one should not "surprise" one's partner by executing an attack that was not previously agreed upon. Self-discipline also includes strict adherence to the training framework, following the session leader's instructions, and a genuine concern for the well-being of one's partner.

Safety Rules and Regulations in Different Fields of Training

The trainee must be prepared, emotionally, physically, and technically, for the level of difficulty inherent in the training session. If, for any reason, one feels that he is unable to handle the confrontation or unable to perform any of the tasks required during the session, **one should refrain from these activities**. The session leader must be aware of the student's abilities and limitations at any given moment, and proceed accordingly.

The practicing of acts such as punches or kicks in the air, should always be done **under appropriate control and with suitable force**, so as not to damage the joints or muscles. A moving limb, for example, must not be released beyond its maximum reach, so as not to harm or overextend the joint. Therefore recoil before your reach full extension.

During the session, the force of impact on the punching bag or any other target, pad, or mitt, shall be **controlled**. The attacking limb must become accustomed to absorbing the shocks received when colliding with the target, and it usually takes some time and training till you can safely hit with high speed and force. It is quite common, in training as well as in real-life incidents, that after succeeding to deliver a punch with his fist, the combatant will suffer injury to his wrist.

In group training, any movement requiring a large space, e.g., falls, fall-breaking, rolls, throws, and kicks, shall be performed **by all participants in the same direction**, in order to avoid collision with each other. **Falling and throwing** must be done onto an appropriately **soft surface**.

If the training place is crowded, actions such as throwing one's partner **should always be coordinated** with the other participants. In such cases, it is also necessary to look in the direction of movement **to avoid possible collision** with other trainees. Under no circumstances shall one student be thrown forcefully in the direction of other participants!

Caution: Unless specifically required, one student should not land forcefully upon his partner at the completion of a takedown, sweep, or throw.

No part of the body, and particularly **no vulnerable point** on the partner's body, shall be subject to powerful attack. We must bear in mind that the possible level of impact in the context of delivering and absorbing an attack differs for every individual. Some people are strong and have a high level of tolerance, while others are more sensitive. However, **forceful attacks to the most vulnerable points on the body almost always result in injury**, sometimes permanent, no matter who is on the receiving end.

Note: The student should never land a punch on his partner's unprotected face with an ungloved fist or with tensed, rigid fingers.

The partner must be released from chokes, headlocks, grabs, or leverage actions **the instant he gives a prearranged signal**, such as uttering a word or a sound, tapping with his hand, etc. This type of attack shall not be performed hurriedly or at maximum force. Instead, these moves must be performed **gradually**, in a controlled manner and with attention to the partner's reactions. Only after one is well-conditioned and has achieved a high level of proficiency in the defense exercises, may a more intense level of training be allowed.

In practicing defenses against attack with a stick, the stick **must be smooth**, with no breaks, cracks, or protrusions. **A padded stick** is recommended in the beginning and during stressful training sessions.

In practicing defenses against knife attack, **rubber knives** should be used in the initial stages of training. Only after an adequate degree of skill has been achieved, may the students progress to dull **wooden knives**. Finally, once they have completely mastered the techniques, the students may train with **metal knives**, but with maximum care!

Note: Training accessories and aids must be kept in good condition, complete, and suitable for the specific activity.

Whenever necessary, the student **shall wear protective gear**, appropriate to his level of physical condition and technical capacities and to the degree of impact in the exercise or encounter. A wide variety of excellent protective gear is available on the market. For your own welfare, you should use protective gear that is appropriate and well designed.

The encounter and the practice session should be stopped immediately if "things get out of hand" and the participants seem to be losing control. This requires that there be **adequate supervision** at the training site. Activity may be resumed only after the trainees have regained emotional, mental, and physical balance and control.

In practicing every technique and confrontation, the partners must be able to trust each other, and must also **help each other achieve their goals**: mastering the exercise and the subject as a whole, improving their skills, and accumulating knowledge. This should be done without the hindrance of destructive competition, the wish to prove superiority, or any attempt to "settle accounts" or seek revenge.

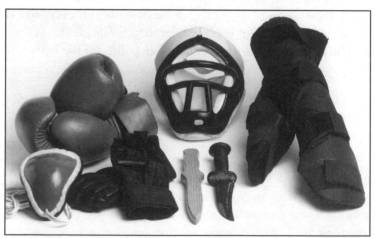

Some safety accessories: Head guard, used mainly in powerful fighting practice; gloves for use with punching bag; regular boxing gloves; shin guards; athletic supporter; wooden and rubber training knives.

Chapter 15

About the Authors

Grandmaster Imi, Founder of Krav Maga

Imi (Imrich) Sde-Or (Lichtenfeld), founder of Krav Maga, was born in 1910 in Budapest, which at the time was one of the centers of the Austro-Hungarian Empire. He grew up in Bratislava, the capital of Slovakia, in a home where sports, abiding by the law, and humanistic education were equally respected. These elements of his upbringing were major factors in the forming of his remarkable character later in life.

Samuel Lichtenfeld, Imi's father, was undoubtedly quite a unique figure. At age 13 he joined a traveling circus, and for the next twenty years engaged in wrestling, weightlifting, and various demonstrations of strength. For him the circus was also a school, where he met people involved in a wide variety of sports, including some very unusual ones. These people taught young Samuel what they knew, including various fighting and self-defense techniques.

After leaving the circus, Samuel Lichtenfeld moved to Bratislava (then known as Presburg) and established the city's first club for heavy athletics, named "**Hercules**" after the mythological Greek hero. He later joined the municipal police department, where he rose to the position of Chief Detective. During his years of service in this post, Samuel gained a reputation as the officer who apprehended and brought to trial

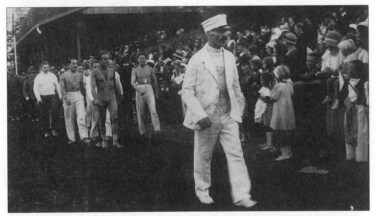

Samuel Lichtenfeld, leading the group (headed by Imi) of Jewish wrestlers adorned with medals, in the Czechoslovakian Independence Day parade.

223

the highest number of murderers and violent criminals.

While serving as a detective, Samuel Lichtenfeld trained his men in self-defense and ways to overcome violent assault, with emphasis on maintaining moral behavior with criminals and upstanding citizens alike. His techniques were highly stylized, perhaps not very effective or overly powerful, but they suited the time, met the needs, and complied with the legal restrictions on police activity during that period.

As a child, Imi was trained by his father in various fields of physical education and sports, including gymnastics, and participated in the training given to the group of detectives that Samuel Lichtenfeld taught regularly. With his father's encouragement, Imi became active in a wide range of sports. He first excelled in swimming, and subsequently in gymnastics, wrestling, and boxing. In 1928 Imi won the Slovakian Youth Wrestling Championship, and in 1929 the adult championship (in the welter-weight division). That year he also won the national boxing championship and an international gymnastics championship.

During the ensuing decade, Imi's athletic activities focused mainly on wrestling, both as a contestant and a trainer. Year after year he won the Slovakian championship for his weight class and was one of the mainstays of the national team. Up until 1939, Imi participated in numerous international meets, winning dozens of medals and prizes. Imi was considered one of the top European wrestlers. He won victories over many champions and title-holders in his own and other countries.

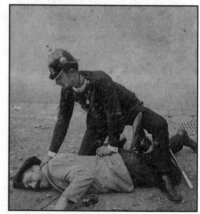

Imi's sports activities also included acrobatics, and from there he branched out into dramatic arts. He taught gymnastics to the cast of one of Czechoslovakia's best-known theater troupes companies, and acted successfully in several of

Samuel Lichtenfeld (as the "criminal") demonstrating with one of his policemen an apprehension and control technique.

its productions. In one of the ballet performances, he played the role of "Mephisto" to the thunderous applause of both the audience and critics.

In the mid-thirties, conditions began to change in Bratislava. Influenced by similar movements in Central Europe, fascist and anti-Semitic factions appeared, determined to upset the public order and harm the city's Jewish community. Imi naturally became the uncrowned leader of a group of young Jews, most of them with a background in boxing, wrestling, and weightlifting. This group of athletes attempted to block the anti-Semitic bands from entering the Jewish quarter and wreaking havoc there.

Thus, between 1936 and 1940 Imi took part in countless violent clashes and street fights with the anti-Semitic thugs, both alone and with his group. He and his companions were often confronted by angry crowds of hundreds and even thousands of people from Bratislava and the surrounding area who tried to enter the Jewish quarter; and sometimes it only was one or two hecklers against Imi or one of his friends, who had to be put in their place. Though space is insufficient to describe the myriad of incidents that occurred during that period, suffice it to say that they molded Imi's mind and body and turned him from a sportsman into a determined hand-to-hand, practical fighter. It was these events that planted in him the seeds that later grew into the self-defense system that he originated, **Krav Maga**.

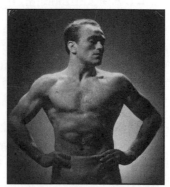

In 1940, having become a thorn in the side of the anti-Semitically inclined local authorities, Imi left his home, family, and friends and boarded the last immigrant ship that succeeded in escaping the Nazis' clutches. The vessel was an ancient riverboat named **Pentcho** that had been converted to carry hundreds of refugees from Central Europe to the promised land of Israel (then called Palestine). The gripping story of the Pentcho and its passengers is told in detail in the book **Odyssey** by John Birman (Simon & Shuster, New York, 1984).

Imi Sde-Or (Lichtenfeld) in his late twenties, at the height of his ability as an outstanding boxer, wrestler, and athlete.

Imi's private odyssey aboard the ship and afterwards, which was filled with thrilling episodes, lasted about two years, until he reached his destination. At the start of his journey, sailing along the Danube River and through the Aegean Sea, Imi had to jump into the water several times to save passengers who had fallen overboard or to retrieve bags of food, which was exceedingly scarce at that time. As a result, he suffered a severe ear infection that nearly cost him his life.

When a boiler exploded on board the ship, causing it to run aground near the Greek island of Kamilanisi, Imi and four friends took a rowboat and set out for Crete to get help. Ignoring his ear infection and the pleas of his friends, Imi refused to relinquish the oars for an entire day. But despite their heroic efforts, strong winds caused the small rowboat to drift, and it never reached Crete. On the morning of the fifth day, a British warship picked up the five survivors and brought them to Alexandria, Egypt. Imi, whose condition had severely deteriorated, was sent to the Jewish hospital in the city, where he underwent a series of operations. It was not until fifty years later that Imi became aware, that he had actually been near death at that time, and the doctors at that hospital had held no hope for his recovery. He learned this when a friend from the rowboat, Joseph Hertz (who later became a physician in Prague), visited Israel.

After recuperating, Imi joined the **Czech Legion**, which was under command of the British Army during World War II. Within this framework, he served for about a year and a half at various points in the Middle East, among them Libya, Egypt, Syria, and Lebanon. Upon his release, in 1942, Imi requested and was granted an entry permit to Israel (then called Palestine).

At that time, several of Imi's friends and former pupils were serving in the **Hagana** resistance, the pre-IDF (Israel Defense Forces) military organization. They introduced Imi to General Itzchak Sadeh, head of the Hagana, who immediately accepted him into the organization in light of his special talents in hand-to-hand combat.

In 1944 Imi began to train Israeli fighters in his areas of expertise: physical fitness, swimming, use of the knife, and defense against knife attacks. During that period, Imi trained several elite units of the **Hagana** and **Palmach** (the renowned striking force of the Hagana and forerunner of the special units of the IDF), including its marine commando unit, the **Palyam**, as well as groups of police officers.

In 1948, coinciding with the birth of the State of Israel and the founding of the Israel Defense Forces, Imi became Chief Instructor for Physical Fitness and Krav Maga at the **School of Combat Fitness**. He served in the IDF for about 20 years, during which time he developed and refined his unique method for self-defense and hand-to-hand combat. Imi personally trained the top fighters of Israel's special units, and qualified many generations of Krav Maga instructors, for which he gained the recognition of Israel's most senior commanders.

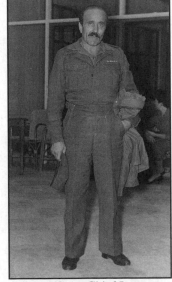

We must bear in mind that Imi's method, Krav Maga, had to meet the varied needs of the IDF. That is, it had to be **easy to learn and apply**, so that the soldier, whether a clerk in an office or a fighter in an elite unit, could attain the required proficiency within the **shortest possible training period**. It was also important, that the soldiers' level of proficiency could be maintained with minimal review and practice. It was even more crucial that the self-defense and fighting techniques that Imi devised could be readily applied under the most stressful conditions.

After retiring from active duty, Imi began adapting Krav Maga to civilian needs. The method was adapted to suit everyone: **man or woman, boy or girl, young people or adults**, anyone who might need it to save his (or her) life and survive an attack, while sustaining minimal harm, whatever the background of attack may be: criminal, nationalistic, or other.

Imi Sde-Or as Chief Instructor of Krav Maga and Physical Training in the Israel Defense Forces.

To disseminate his method, Imi established two training centers, in Tel Aviv and Netanya, his home town. Incidentally Netanya, this fascinating Mediterranean tourist resort where many of top Krav Maga instructors came from, quickly became known as a pilgrimage site for ardent disciples of this original Israeli fighting system.

Throughout that time, Imi Sde-Or continued to serve as a consultant and Krav Maga instructor for the IDF as well as other Israeli security forces. In 1972 the first civilian course for Krav Maga instructors was held at the School for Trainers and Instructors at the **Wingate Institute of Sport and Physical Education**. Since then, the method has spread to numerous civilian frameworks in Israel and abroad.

Many thousands of people have been trained in the easy-to-grasp, no-nonsense self-defense techniques of Krav Maga. Besides members of the Israeli security services and the Israeli Police, it is taught in teachers' colleges, elementary schools, private institutes, as well as in private studios, rural settlements (such as **kibbutzim** and **moshavim**) and in local urban community centers.

In 1978, Imi and some of his most devoted students founded the **Israeli Krav Maga Association**, intended to disseminate the method in Israel and abroad and impart its values of self-defense. Imi Sde-Or served as President of the Association for life.

International activity began in 1981, mainly in the United States, with the generous assistance of the American publicly spirited businessman Mr. Daniel Abraham. The successful spreading of Krav Maga teaching in the US was mainly due to the energetic activity of Mr. Darren R. Levine (Master Level 1/Expert level 6) of Los Angeles, California. Since the eighties, Mr. Levine has been laboring to introduce Imi's self-defense method to the American public and also contribute to the English-language edition of this book as its Technical Adviser and Professional Editor.

In the early nineties, Grandmaster Imi expressed his wish to establish an **International Krav Maga Federation**, aiming to spread his special knowledge to people worldwide. Eventually founded, it was warmly welcomed by Imi, who viewed it as his life's dream coming true. In 1996 Imi awarded Eyal Yanilov, the originator and Head Instructor of the Federation (and co-author of this book), the ultimate rank of Master level 3/Expert level 8 for all of his accomplishments.

Until his very last days, at eighty-seven years of age, Imi continued, assisted by Eyal Yanilov, to develop Krav Maga techniques and concepts. He personally supervised the training of those with the highest rankings in Krav Maga and spent time with instructors in Israel and those visiting from abroad. Imi monitored the trainees' progress and achievements, captivating them with his unique personality and his sharp sense of humor and imparting them with his knowledge and advice.

Grandmaster Imi Sde-Or passed away in January 1998, maintaining good spirits even in his final moments, knowing that his teaching is alive and flourishing.

Eyal Yanilov

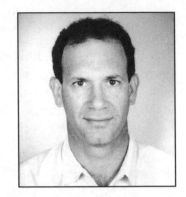

Eyal Yanilov (born 1959) studied Krav Maga under the personal tutelage of its founder, Imi Sde-Or (Lichtenfeld), and served as the Grandmaster's closest assistant and foremost disciple since the early 1980s. Active in this field since 1973, he is now its most senior instructor. Mr. Yanilov is the only individual who holds the highest rank ever given by Imi (Master level 3/Expert level 8), as well as the unique "Founder's Diploma of Excellence," which is held only by Mr. Yanilov and Mr. Darren Levine of the United States.

Eyal Yanilov started his Krav Maga training with Mr. Eli Avikzar (one of Imi's top students) and soon afterwards began to study directly under the founder himself. At an early age, Eyal was instructing at the training studio in Netanya that Imi had entrusted to Eli Avikzar, and on many occasions assisted and substituted for the Grandmaster in lessons and preparations with students who were to be tested for grades of expert level. At a later stage, when Imi appointed him Head of the Krav Maga Professional Committee, Eyal was responsible for preparing and updating the Krav Maga curriculum. In this capacity Eyal had the task of imparting the new developments and accumulated knowledge, changes in techniques, and the latest training methods to the other senior instructors.

In 1984 Grandmaster Imi Sde-Or placed Eyal in charge of preparing the complete and comprehensive series of books on the Krav Maga discipline (of which this volume is a part). Since then, and until the system's founder passed away in 1998, the two were deeply engrossed in the task of writing down the principles of Krav Maga and clarifying its various techniques.

Since directing the first self-defense instructors course for American citizens in 1981, Eyal Yanilov has taught a large number of Krav Maga and self-defense instructors courses in many countries around the world, under the auspices of the Israeli Krav Maga Association, Israel's Ministry of Education, and the International Krav Maga Federation (IKMF). He, and his most advanced students who serve as local directors or chief instructors in their countries, are the key force in spreading Krav Maga teaching throughout the world. Mr. Yanilov is currently serving as Chairman and Chief Instructor of the IKMF*, and heads the **International School of Krav Maga**. In this capacity, he is in charge of the development, definition, and dissemination of the system worldwide.

Mr. Yanilov is a graduate of the School for Trainers and Instructors at the **Wingate Institute for Sport and Physical Education**, and also holds a degree in Electrical Engineering. He has spent years training fighters of Israeli and foreign elite units and members of special anti-terrorist squads, while also teaching Krav Maga at colleges for physical education teachers.

Since the early eighties Eyal has been training various groups, in a variety of seminars and courses, including ordinary civilians coming to learn self-defense, military units, police units, executive protection personnel, special units, SWAT teams, and other security-oriented groups in Israel, Europe, South America, the United States, Australia, New Zealand, and Japan. Within this context, he specializes in improving the fighting skills and general abilities of members of these groups. Mr. Yanilov's main objective now is to educate future KM instructors around the world, to spread the knowledge of Krav Maga in their native countries, and he always enjoys promoting any initiative in this direction.

*IKMF & International Scool of Krav Maga: P.O. Box 2661, Netanya 42126, Israel; **Fax**: +972-9-8910863, and on the web: **www.krav-maga.com**.

Editor: Darren Levine

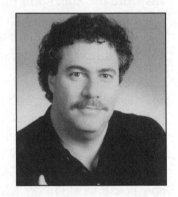

Darren R. Levine (born 1960) is Chief Executive Officer and Chief Instructor of the Krav Maga National Training Center* in Los Angeles, California. Mr. Levine is the highest-ranking Krav Maga instructor in the United States. In 1981, Mr. Levine participated in the first International Krav Maga Instructors Course offered to candidates from outside Israel, sponsored by the Israeli Ministry of Education and supervised by Grandmaster Imi Sde-Or (Lichtenfeld).

Mr. Levine was taught by Grandmaster Imi, by Eyal Yanilov, and by other leading civilian and military instructors of Krav Maga. He was awarded his first Expert Degree (Black Belt) in 1983, his Full Instructor's Degree (from the Wingate Institute of Physical Education and Sport) in 1984, and his Master Level 1 (6th Degree Black Belt) in December 1997. Darren is one of the top Krav Maga instructors in the world, and is also among those select individuals who hold the highest ranks; he is one of only two individuals who hold the Founder's Diploma of Excellence.

Mr. Levine has taught self-defense and fighting applications of Krav Maga in the US to thousands of civilians of all ages. In addition, he has taught Krav Maga extensively to US local, state, and federal law-enforcement agencies, including special operations and anti-terrorist units.

Because of his astute understanding of both Krav Maga and the specific needs of law-enforcement personnel, particularly in the US, Mr. Levine developed the basic law-enforcement Krav Maga curriculum in the US. Additionally, he has made significant contributions to the growth and spread of Krav Maga among civilians in the United States.

In addition to Mr. Levine's Krav Maga-related work, he serves as a Senior Deputy District Attorney for the County of Los Angeles. Mr. Levine is assigned to the Special Operations Division, where he is responsible for prosecuting serious and violent crimes committed against peace officers.

*Krav Maga National Training Center, Los Angeles, California,
  Tel. (310) 966-1300, and on the web: www.kravmaga.com.

Publisher: Zvi Morik

Zvi D. Morik (born 1947) began learning Krav Maga in 1967, directly under its founder, Imi Sde-Or. He first became acquainted with Grandmaster Imi at the training studio that he opened for civilians near Dizengoff Square, Tel Aviv. In the following years, Zvi was Imi's disciple, and then his close assistant and personal friend for over thirty years, until the Grandmaster passed away. As a young man, Zvi was deeply impressed by Imi's remarkable characteristics as an educator, a Martial Arts expert and an exceptional human being, and was immediately captivated by his outstanding, radiant personality.

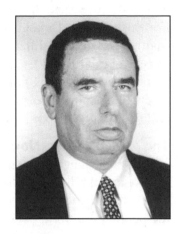

Throughout his university years, Zvi improved his knowledge of Krav Maga, enjoying the privilege of studying under the Grandmaster's personal tutelage, which was indeed unparalleled (and also with his senior assistant-instructor at the time, Eli Avikzar). Twenty years later, when Eyal Yanilov, Imi's foremost disciple, opened his Krav Maga classes in Tel Aviv, Zvi resumed his training under Eyal's instruction.

After Zvi Morik received his university degree (in Mathematics, Statistics and Economics), Imi Sde-Or chose him to serve as his assistant in building the Krav Maga organization. In 1978, he was one of the few founders of the **Israeli Krav Maga Association**, serving as its first General Secretary and later as its Spokesman and PR Director. For his devotion in carrying out these roles, Zvi was later awarded an Honorary Black Belt by the Association.

Shortly after Zvi Morik established his publishing company, **Dekel Academic Press**, and became a professional publisher, Grandmaster Imi asked him to undertake the entire editing and publishing activity of the Krav Maga publications in Israel and abroad, an obligation that he readily accepted. It should be noted that since the mid-eighties, the various techniques of the Krav Maga discipline have been systematically organized, mainly under the direction of Eyal Yanilov, who later also co-authored this series with Imi Sde-Or. In 1990 Zvi Morik published a first outline of the Krav Maga series in English, in the form of an abstract under the **Tamar Books** imprint. This was followed in 1992 with a Hebrew-language publication entitled: *How to Defend Yourself against Knife Attacks* by Imi Sde-Or and Eyal Yanilov. The late Mr. Yitzhak Rabin, then Israel's Prime Minister, and previously the Israel Defense Forces' Chief of Staff, who knew Imi and respected his educational activity as Chief Instructor of Krav Maga at the army, honored his book by writing a foreword.

During this period, Zvi, who had become Imi's personal adviser and one of his closest friends, indefatigably strived to fulfill his teacher's dream that Krav Maga knowledge would be accessible the world over to anybody who may need it in time of danger. For this purpose, Dekel was transformed into an international publishing company (named Dekel Publishing House*, incorporating both its imprints, Dekel Academic Press & Tamar Books), and Zvi Morik began taking part in central publishing events and international book fairs. Together with several of his colleagues, he established a new publishing association, **the Israel Publishers' Union**, was named its president, and is currently responsible for the Union's international relations.

The present volume, *How to Defend Yourself against Armed Assault,* is the result of a co-publishing venture that was established in mid-1999 between **Dekel Publishing House** and the US publisher **Frog Ltd**. In the near future this book is scheduled to be translated and published in several other languages as well, for the benefit of all the people, the world over, who are interested in Karv Maga.

***Dekel Publising House**, P.O. Box 45094, Tel Aviv 61450, Israel;
 Fax: +972-3-5273011, and on the web: **www.dekelpublishing.com**

Concepts and Terms Commonly Used in Krav Maga

This chapter presents concepts and terms commonly used in Krav Maga, which appear in this book.

Outlet Stances

Outlet stance: Starting position, from which the various defenses and attacks are performed.

Neutral outlet stance: Straight body, hands down, and feet parallel and shoulder-width apart. Often referred to as "**passive stance**." It serves to simulate a person's natural stance, when he is not particularly braced for possibly being attacked.

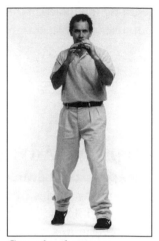
General outlet stance.

General outlet stance: Often referred to as a "general fighting stance." The placement of the feet falls between standing in an astride position with the feet shoulder-width apart) and a linear position, when one foot is directly behind the other with a space of about 6-13 inches (15-33cm) between them. The heel of the rear foot is raised, the knees are slightly bent, the forward foot is turned slightly inward, and the hands are raised to shoulder or neck height with each hand placed opposite the inner side of the corresponding shoulder and at an equal distance from it. A half to two-thirds of the body weight is on the forward foot.

Note: This is just a general formula for an outlet stance; each individual may change it slightly and adapt it to suit himself or herself, especially during a confrontation.

Outlet stance for inside defenses: As above, except that the horizontal distance between the hands is slightly greater, and each hand is approximately opposite the corresponding shoulder.

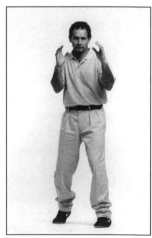
Outlet stance for inside defenses.

Objective: Mainly used for maximum comfort while

learning and practicing the techniques that utilize inside defenses against straight punches. Also, this position draws the attack to the center, between the defender's hands, facilitating an easier defense.

Outlet stance for outside defenses: Similar to the general outlet stance, except that each hand is in front of the opposite shoulder and the body can be turned slightly.

Objective: Used mainly for maximum comfort while learning and practicing the techniques that utilize outside defenses against straight punches.

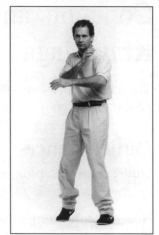

Outlet stance for outside defenses.

Steps and Advancing Technique

Stomping step, advancing by stomping step: Advancing technique from a neutral position, by means of a low bursting step, advancing (with a skip) on one foot, usually while the other foot or leg delivers a kick. The forward foot can also be advanced in this way, from the general outlet stance (see above).

Crossing, advancing by crossing: Advancing by a low bursting step (using a skip) forward, while crossing your legs in order to gain proper distance and range. This is accomplished with motions similar to the stomping step described above. When the rear foot passes in front of the forward foot, the action is called "forward crossing," and when it passes behind the forward foot, the action is called "backward crossing." When the advancing foot lands, the other foot is already in the air, on its way to the target, executing a kick or a knee.

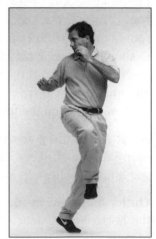

Advancing by backward crossing.

Pursuing step: Also a member of the family of stomping steps. Rapid advance in which the rear foot advances and replaces the forward one. The moment the advancing leg touches the ground, the other (usually the front) leg is on its way to hit the target.

Punches

Straight punch: A punch in which the hand is sent in a straight line from the shoulder area to the target, and the elbow is low for as long as possible. When the punch is near completion, the fist rotates slightly, and then the hand recoils immediately in a powerful movement, resembling a backward "pumping" action. This springlike recoiling motion, executed in most punches in Krav Maga, increases the speed of the punch, resulting in a stronger concussion on impact with the target. The punch is usually executed with the heel of the hand or with a clenched fist, striking the target with the knuckles of the index and middle fingers.

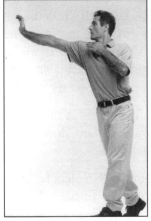

Straight right punch with the heel of the hand.

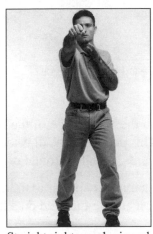

Straight right punch viewed from the front.

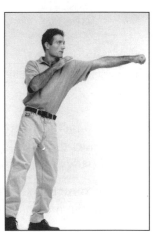

Straight left punch.

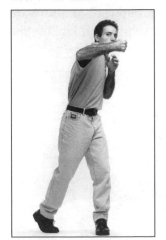

Roundhouse "hook" punch with the right hand.

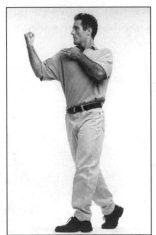

Uppercut punch with the right hand.

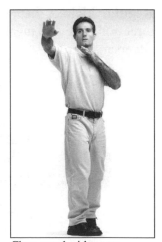

Chop punch sideways.

Roundhouse "hook" punch: The fist is delivered forward in a semicircular, inward movement designed to go around any obstacle on its way to the target. The body

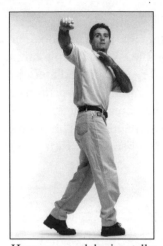
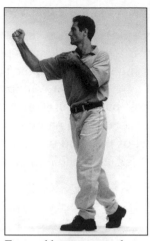

Hammer punch horizontally backwards.

Forward hammer punch.

pivots in the direction of the attack, with the attacker's weight applied to the punch. The fist is held here with the pinkie down and the thumb up, with the knuckles of the index and middle fingers striking the target.

Uppercut punch: The fist advances upward towards the target, generally in a diagonally forward motion. The attacker's body, with all its weight, shoots up sharply upon delivering this punch.

Chop: A punch delivered with the inner edge of the hand. The target is hit by the muscle under the little finger. This punch can be directed forward, inward, downward, outward (sideways), or backwards, on a horizontal or vertical plane.

Hammer punch: Executed in a manner similar to the chop, but with a clenched fist. Similar to the previous punch, it can be directed on a horizontal or vertical plane.

Kicks

Regular kick: A snapping kick that reaches its target in an upward and forward direction. The striking area is the ball of the foot or the instep (when kicking the adversary's groin).

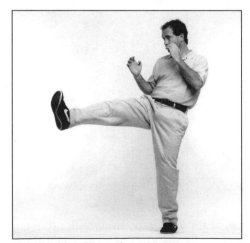
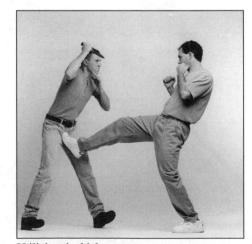

Regular kick forwards.

Utilizing the kick.

Roundhouse kick: A snapping or sweeping kick, coming at the target in a semicircular movement. While performing this action, the kicker executes a pelvic turn. Impact can be made using the ball of the foot, the instep, or sometimes the shinbone (when one is relatively close to the target).

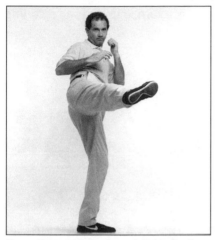

Roundhouse kick, viewed from the front.

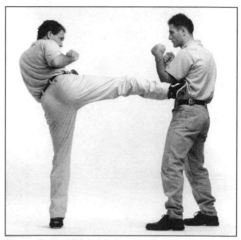

Roundhouse kick hitting the lower ribs.

Stomping kick: This attack is a straight one, hitting the target in a straight line. The foot is lifted and the heel is dropped in a sharp downward movement (as if to flatten a soda can on the ground). The kicker brings his knee up (towards the body) and then sends his heel straight down and towards the target, applying substantial weight. This kick is recoiled quickly and can be directed downward (stomp), forward (defensive kick forward), sideways (side kick) or backwards (defensive back kick).

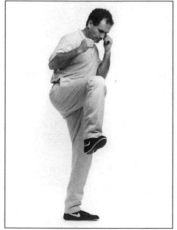

Raising the knee to deliver a downward stomping kick.

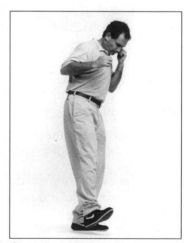

Stomping down.

Side kick: The kick is generally delivered to a target located to the kicker's side. This is a variation of the stomping kick. The kicker brings his knee up and forward, pivoting on the hip joint. This brings the foot lateral to the target. The heel is sent to the target in a straight thrusting movement. The hip of the kicking leg moves towards the target as the base foot pivots for greater extension, and the body leans slightly to the side. After delivering the kick, the foot is returned in a strong recoiling motion, virtually along the same path that it was sent.

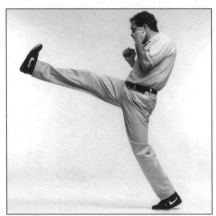

Defensive kick forward.

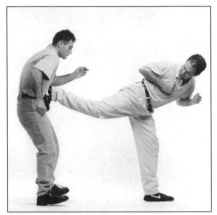

Defensive kick backwards.

Defensive back kick: This kick also belongs to the family of stomping kicks. The heel is sent from near the buttocks in a straight line towards the target, similar to the way a horse kicks with its hind leg. The back is curved, and in order to see the target, the kicker looks backwards, beside his shoulder or under his arm.

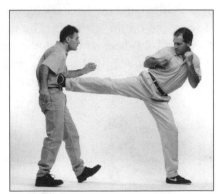

Side kick.

Defenses

Outside defense: An action that deflects or stops the attack. From near the body, the defending limb (e.g., the forearm) is sent out to the outside, up, or down.

Inside defense: An action that deflects (or stops) the attack. The defending limb moves in to meet the attack, and redirects it by crossing the path of the attacking limb at a right or acute angle.

"Stabbing" defense: An outside defense that meets the attacking limb at an acute angle and slides along it, thereby diverting it from its course. This technique is characterized by linear movement, similar to the straight punch.

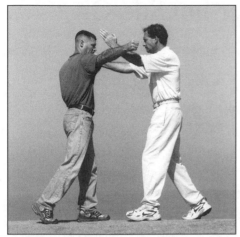

Outside defense against a straight punch.

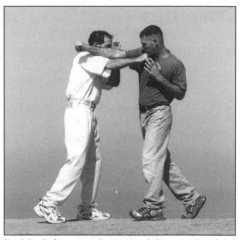

Inside defense against a straight punch with a simultaneous counterattack.

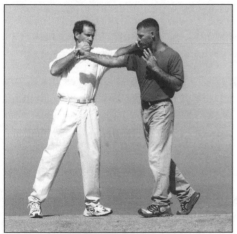

Inside sliding defense, hitting at the end of the defensive move.

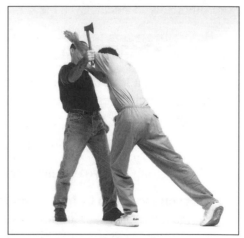

Stabbing defense against an attack with an ax.

Hand Movements

Supination: A rotating movement of the forearm and hand on an axis that is parallel to the forearm, sending the thumb to the outside. The right hand moves clockwise and the left, counterclockwise.

Leverage: Bending any joint beyond its natural limit in order to apply pressure to it and to cause the adversary pain, possibly dislocate the joint, control it in its present position, or cause the adversary to move in the direction dictated by the defender.

Cavalier: Wrist bend plus supination, creating a powerful leverage action that immediately drops the adversary to the ground.

Sayings of Grandmaster Imi Sde-Or

- He whose "NO" is not a real NO, neither is his "YES" a real YES.

- Tell people the truth and they will "give it to you" right in the face.

- One need not make peace with friends, only with enemies...

- Strict reckoning keeps good friendship.

- A strong man always has many friends.

- Not everyone who walks on two legs is indeed a human being.

- He who signs his name in capital letters, is not a man.

- There are no two things in life that are exactly the same. Even twin brothers slightly differ. Even two screws that come off the same assembly line are not completely identical. Even the same person may be different at different moments.

- Before beginning to court a woman, you would better know who her father is, who her brothers are, and sometimes even who her boyfriend is...

- Sometimes a man turns his head to look at a woman and it changes his entire life, and sometimes he does not turn his head and that, too, completely changes his life.

- I do not travel abroad in order to see the sights; I go only to meet people.

- Waiter, bring me two of whatever my doctors do not allow me to have!

- **Everyone wants to be in someone else's place**: At the circus a young, muscular gymnast performs acrobatic feats on the trapeze, while in the audience below, in the most expensive seat, sits a rich, fat businessman with a cigar between his lips and a stunning girl on his arm. The businessman says to himself: "I would give all I have in order to be like him, young, athletic, without a care in the world," and the acrobat, who sees him from high up on the trapeze, thinks: "I wish I could be in his place, a rich man with such a beautiful woman, who can afford the most expensive seat at the circus and watch a young, poor, unfortunate guy like me endanger his life for a few cents."